Gastroenterology

Editor

JENNIFER R. EAMES

PHYSICIAN ASSISTANT CLINICS

www.physicianassistant.theclinics.com

Consulting Editor
JAMES A. VAN RHEE

October 2021 • Volume 6 • Number 4

ELSEVIER

1600 John F. Kennedy Boulevard • Suite 1800 • Philadelphia, Pennsylvania, 19103-2899

http://www.theclinics.com

PHYSICIAN ASSISTANT CLINICS Volume 6, Number 4
October 2021 ISSN 2405-7991, ISBN-13: 978-0-323-79426-8

Editor: Katerina Heidhausen
Developmental Editor: Axell Ivan Jade Purificacion

Physician Assistant Clinics (ISSN: 2405–7991) is published quarterly by Elsevier Inc., 360 Park Avenue South, New York, NY 10010-1710. Months of issue are January, April, July, and October. Periodicals postage paid at New York, NY and additional mailing offices. Subscription prices are $150.00 per year (US individuals), $290.00 (US institutions), $100.00 (US students), $150.00 (Canadian individuals), $297.00 (Canadian institutions), $100.00 (Canadian students), $150.00 (international individuals), $297.00 (international institutions), and $100.00 (international students). Foreign air speed delivery is included in all *Clinics* subscription prices. All prices are subject to change without notice. POSTMASTER: Send address changes to *Physician Assistant Clinics*, Elsevier Periodicals Customer Service, 11830 Westline Industrial Drive, St. Louis, MO 63146. Customer Service Health Sciences Division, Subscription Customer Service, 3251 Riverport Lane, Maryland Heights, MO 63043. **Customer Service: 1-800-654-2452 (U.S. and Canada); 314-447-8871 (outside U.S. and Canada). Fax: 314-447-8029. E-mail: journalscustomerservice-usa@elsevier.com (for print support); journalsonlinesupport-usa@elsevier.com (for online support).**

Reprints. For copies of 100 or more, of articles in this publication, please contact the Commercial Reprints Department, Elsevier Inc., 360 Park Avenue South, New York, NY 10010-1710. Tel. 212-633-3874; Fax: 212-633-3820; E-mail: reprints@elsevier.com.

Physician Assistant Clinics is covered in *EMBASE/Excerpta Medica* and *ESCI*.

PROGRAM OBJECTIVE
The goal of the Physician Assistant Clinics is to keep practicing physician assistants up to date with current clinical practice by providing timely articles reviewing the state of the art in patient care.

TARGET AUDIENCE
Physician Assistants and other healthcare professionals

LEARNING OBJECTIVES
Upon completion of this activity, participants will be able to:
1. Review updated guidelines for screening and treatment of GI & liver disorders.
2. Discuss best practices in the management of complex GI disorders.
3. Recognize the latest information regarding nutritional deficiencies, supplements, and dietary trends.

ACCREDITATION
The Elsevier Office of Continuing Medical Education (EOCME) is accredited by the Accreditation Council for Continuing Medical Education (ACCME) to provide continuing medical education for physicians.

The EOCME designates this journal-based CME activity for a maximum of 11 *AMA PRA Category 1 Credit*(s)™. Physicians should claim only the credit commensurate with the extent of their participation in the activity.

All other healthcare professionals requesting continuing education credit for this enduring material will be issued a certificate of participation.

DISCLOSURE OF CONFLICTS OF INTEREST
The EOCME assesses conflict of interest with its instructors, faculty, planners, and other individuals who are in a position to control the content of CME activities. All relevant conflicts of interest that are identified are thoroughly vetted by EOCME for fair balance, scientific objectivity, and patient care recommendations. EOCME is committed to providing its learners with CME activities that promote improvements or quality in healthcare and not a specific proprietary business or a commercial interest.

The planning committee, staff, authors and editors listed below have identified no financial relationships or relationships to products or devices they or their spouse/life partner have with commercial interest related to the content of this CME activity:
Shane Ryan Apperley, MSc, PGCert, PA-R; Esther Bennitta; Michael Bessette, MD; Tina M. Butler, DMSc, MPAS, PA-C; Regina Chavous-Gibson, MSN, RN; Jennifer R. Eames, MPAS, DHSc, PA-C; Jennifer Hastings, MSHS, PA-C; Helen Martin, DHSc, PA-C, DFAAPA; Matthew J. McDonald, MS, PA-C; Paula Miksa, DMS, EdS, MHS, PA-C; Kathy J. Robinson, DHSc, MPAS, PA-C; Elisabeth J. Shell, MPAS, PhD, PA-C; Bau Tran, MMS, PharmD, PA-C; James A. Van Rhee, MS, PA-C; Tenell Zahodnik, MPAS, PA-C, CAQ-EM

The planning committee, staff, authors and editors listed below have identified financial relationships or relationships to products or devices they or their spouse/life partner have with commercial interest related to the content of this CME activity:
Amy Kassebaum-Ladewski, PA-C, RD, MMS: Consultant/Advisor: Ironwood Pharmaceuticals, Inc., Salix Pharmaceuticals, Alfasigma USA, Inc.

UNAPPROVED/OFF-LABEL USE DISCLOSURE
The EOCME requires CME faculty to disclose to the participants:
1. When products or procedures being discussed are off-label, unlabelled, experimental, and/or investigational (not US Food and Drug Administration [FDA] approved); and
2. Any limitations on the information presented, such as data that are preliminary or that represent ongoing research, interim analyses, and/or unsupported opinions. Faculty may discuss information about pharmaceutical agents that is outside of FDA-approved labelling. This information is intended solely for CME and is not intended to promote off-label use of these medications. If you have any questions, contact the medical affairs department of the manufacturer for the most recent prescribing information.

TO ENROLL
The CME program is available to all Physician Assistant Clinics subscribers at no additional fee. To subscribe to the Physician Assistant Clinics, call customer service at 1-800-654-2452 or sign up online at www.physicianassistant.theclinics.com/.

METHOD OF PARTICIPATION

In order to claim credit, participants must complete the following:

1. Complete enrolment as indicated above
2. Read the activity
3. Complete the CME Test and Evaluation. Participants must achieve a score of 70% on the test. All CME Tests and Evaluations must be completed online

CME INQUIRIES/SPECIAL NEEDS

For all CME inquiries or special needs, please contact elsevierCME@elsevier.com.

Contributors

CONSULTING EDITOR

JAMES A. VAN RHEE, MS, PA-C
Associate Professor, Program Director, Yale School of Medicine, Yale Physician Assistant Online Program, New Haven, Connecticut

EDITOR

JENNIFER R. EAMES, MPAS, DHSc, PA-C
Program Director and Associate Professor, Physician Assistant Department, Hardin-Simmons University, Abilene, Texas

AUTHORS

SHANE RYAN APPERLEY, MSc, PGCert PA-R
Associate Professor and Director of Didactic Education, PA Program, Lincoln Memorial University, Harrogate, Tennessee

MICHAEL BESSETTE, MD
Assistant Clinical Professor, Physician Assistant Program, Bouvé College, Northeastern University, Boston, Massachusetts

TINA M. BUTLER, DMSc, MPAS, PA-C
Associate Program Director, Assistant Professor, Hardin-Simmons University Physician Assistant Program, Abilene, Texas

JENNIFER R. EAMES, MPAS, DHSc, PA-C
Program Director and Associate Professor, Physician Assistant Department, Hardin-Simmons University, Abilene, Texas

JENNIFER HASTINGS, MSHS, PA-C
Niceville, Florida

AMY KASSEBAUM-LADEWSKI, PA-C, RD, MMS
Digestive Health Center, Northwestern Memorial Hospital, Chicago, Illinois

HELEN MARTIN, DHSC, PA-C, DFAAPA
Division Director of Master of Science in Physician Assistant Studies, Charleston, South Carolina

MATTHEW J. McDONALD, MS, PA-C
Assistant Professor, School of Physician Assistant Studies, Massachusetts College of Pharmacy and Health Sciences University, Boston, Massachusetts

PAULA MIKSA, DMS, EdS, MHS, PA-C
Assistant Dean and Program Director, Doctor of Medical Science (DMS) Program, Lincoln Memorial University, Harrogate, Tennessee

KATHY J. ROBINSON, DHSc, MPAS, PA-C
Hardin-Simmons University, Physician Assistant Program, Abilene, Texas

ELISABETH J. SHELL, MPAS, PhD, PA-C
Assistant Professor, Physician Assistant Program, Baylor College of Medicine, Houston, Texas

BAU TRAN, MMS, PharmD, PA-C
Assistant Professor, UT Southwestern Department of Physician Assistant Studies, Clinical Associate Professor, Texas Tech University College of Pharmacy, Dallas, Texas

TENELL ZAHODNIK, MPAS, PA-C, CAQ-EM
Adjunct Faculty of Emergency Medicine, Department of Physician Assistant Studies, Hardin-Simmons University, Abilene, Texas

Contents

Foreword: Gastroenterology Issue   xi

James A. Van Rhee

Preface: Gastroenterology for Physician Assistants Today   xiii

Jennifer R. Eames

Hepatitis C: Cure for a New Era   555

Jennifer R. Eames and Bau Tran

> Hepatitis C has a huge global impact on mortality and morbidity because it can lead to cirrhosis and liver cancer. Recent recommendations on screening patients may help identify more patients for treatment in a timely manner. New oral direct-acting antiviral therapies have high cure rates with low side effect profiles. To reach the goal of eradication additional clinicians need to be aware of hepatitis C risk factors, screening, and treatment protocols to meet the global demand for care. Physician assistants and providers in primary care can be safe and effective partners in care for the eradication of hepatitis C.

Review of Celiac Disease: Clinical Manifestations, Diagnosis, and Management   569

Helen Martin

> Celiac disease is an autoimmune disease that is characterized by a gastrointestinal response in genetically susceptible persons to dietary gluten causing small intestinal injury. Celiac disease is usually resolved by a gluten-free diet. Despite an increased awareness and improvement in diagnostic testing, most individuals with celiac disease still remain undiagnosed. This article reviews the current literature regarding manifestations, genetic diagnostic testing, and management of celiac disease. Clinicians continue to strive for a better understanding of this disease, patient challenges, and treatments options, which thereby enhances patient outcomes.

Evaluating Patients for Nutritional Deficiencies   581

Tenell Zahodnik

> Linus Pauling said, "Optimum nutrition is the medicine of tomorrow." The phrase nutritional deficiency is an umbrella over an array of complications that affects billions across the globe. These deficiencies can cause a wide scope of health complications, which have the potential to affect every system of the body. This work reviews the diagnosis, evaluation, and management of common nutritional deficiencies, including those related to vitamins A, B1, B3, B9, B12, C, and D and iron. Special populations are reviewed related to these disorders including patients with alcohol use

disorders, celiac disease, post–bariatric surgery, Down syndrome, and the elderly.

Eosinophilic Esophagitis: An Emerging Disorder for Co-management   593

Kathy J. Robinson

Eosinophilic esophagitis (EoE) is a common disease among adults and children that can cause dysphagia and food impaction. Physician assistants (PAs) play a key role in identifying the disease through history, physical examination, and referral for evaluation by a gastroenterologist, allergist, otolaryngologist, pathologist, and dietician as needed. With the care coordination among gastroenterologists, allergists, pediatricians, otolaryngologists, and pathologists, PAs can play a role in early detection and improved quality of life for patients with EoE.

Pathophysiology of Peptic Ulcer Disease   603

Elisabeth J. Shell

Peptic ulcer disease (PUD) is characterized by an imbalance of protective and damaging mechanisms in the upper digestive tract. The cause of PUD was initially thought to be the result of gastric acid hypersecretion, dietary factors, and/or stress. However, Helicobacter pylori infection and nonsteroidal antiinflammatory drugs are now considered the main cause of ulcer formation in the stomach and duodenum.

Refractory Gastroesophageal Reflux Disease: A Closer Look   613

Jennifer Hastings

Gastroesophageal reflux disease (GERD) is a common complaint in both the primary care and specialty settings. Patients often present with persistent symptoms despite treatment with proton-pump inhibitors, prompting additional testing, specialty referrals, and different therapeutic regimens. Refractory GERD presents many management challenges. This guide focuses on an approach to refractory GERD, touching on the importance of lifestyle and dietary modifications, medication optimization, indications and utility of diagnostic testing modalities, and an overview of antireflux procedures.

Updated Screening Strategies for Colorectal Cancer   625

Tina M. Butler

Colorectal cancer (CRC) is the third leading cause of cancer-related death in men and women. Rates of CRC screening for average-risk adults has recently improved but unfortunately, they are not at the recommended goal. Multiple societies have published CRC screening guidelines, but their lack of concordance creates confusion for providers and patients. Improving awareness about CRC screening guidelines and using interventions to overcome barriers can improve screening rates and save lives.

Irritable Bowel Syndrome–Strategies for Diagnosis and Management 637

Amy Kassebaum-Ladewski

Irritable bowel syndrome is a chronic relapsing brain-gut disorder characterized by abdominal pain associated with altered defecation. Using the diagnostic criteria for IBS and ruling out the presence of alarm signs and symptoms, a confident diagnosis of IBS can be made without superfluous testing. Our understanding of the pathophysiology of IBS continues to evolve and includes factors such as visceral hypersensitivity, alterations in gut-brain interactions, dysbiosis, bile-acid malabsorption, and enteric infections. Consequently, treatment for IBS is not one-size-fits-all. Recognizing the interplay and evidence supporting dietary, behavioral, and pharmaceutical interventions is imperative to providing effective comprehensive care.

Inflammatory Bowel Disease: Managing Complex Patients 655

Paula Miksa and Shane Ryan Apperley

Inflammatory bowel disease is a disorder of the gastrointestinal tract, classified as either Crohn disease (CD) or ulcerative colitis (UC). Both conditions have unknown cause and are often difficult to diagnose and treat. The management of patients with CD or UC typically involves multiple health care personnel and the combination of lifestyle changes, medical pharmacotherapy, and surgical intervention. Special patient groups, namely children, the elderly, and women who are pregnant or breastfeeding, each have their own unique management considerations that must be recognized and addressed.

Nonalcoholic Fatty Liver Disease: The New Epidemic 667

Michael Bessette

Nonalcoholic fatty liver disease (NAFLD) is becoming the leading cause of chronic liver disease and cirrhosis worldwide. Triglyceride deposition in the liver without other causes, including excess alcohol intake, is diagnostic. Those with obesity or insulin resistance should be screened using the Fatty Liver Index (FLI). Imaging can confirm the presence of hepatic steatosis. Inflammation may lead to fibrosis, cirrhosis, or primary liver cancer. NALFD patients should be screened using FIB-4 for referral to elastography or biopsy. Treatment includes a Mediterranean diet and regular exercise. Metformin and statins alone will not improve NAFLD. Bariatric surgery and liver transplant are options.

Acute Gastrointestinal Bleeding – Locating the Source and Correcting the Disorder 677

Matthew J. McDonald

In the United States, gastrointestinal (GI) bleeding is a common medical condition in both emergency and outpatient settings. This article will serve as a review of current management and practice guidelines on the approach to treating nonvariceal acute upper GI bleeding, small bowel bleeding, and acute lower GI bleeding.

PHYSICIAN ASSISTANT CLINICS

FORTHCOMING ISSUES

January 2022
Preventive Medicine
Stephanie Neary, *Editor*

April 2022
The Kidney
Kim Zuber and Jane S. Davis, *Editors*

July 2022
Obstetrics and Gynecology
Elyse Watkins, *Editor*

RECENT ISSUES

July 2021
Behavioral Health
Kim Zuber and Jane S. Davis, *Editors*

April 2021
Surgery
Courtney Fankhanel, *Editor*

January 2021
Rheumatology
Benjamin J Smith, *Editor*

SERIES OF RELATED INTEREST

Psychiatric Clinics
https://www.psych.theclinics.com/

THE CLINICS ARE AVAILABLE ONLINE!
Access your subscription at:
www.theclinics.com

Foreword

Gastroenterology Issue

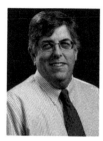

James A. Van Rhee, MS, PA-C
Consulting Editor

Gastrointestinal disorders, such as diarrhea, nausea, vomiting, abdominal pain, jaundice, or rectal bleeding, are commonly seen by physician assistants. According to the National Ambulatory Medical Care Survey, in 2018, there were over 37.2 million physician office visits resulting in a primary diagnosis of digestive disease.[1] Stomach or abdominal pain made up 9.4 million office visits and gastroesophageal reflux disease made up 7.5 million cases in 2018.[1] In 2014, digestive disease was the primary diagnosis in 15.7 million emergency department visits.[2] The most common diagnoses in the emergency department were abdominal pain with 6 million diagnoses, nausea/vomiting with 2.1 million diagnoses, and noninfectious gastroenteritis/colitis with 1.2 million diagnoses.[2]

As you can see from these numbers, physician assistants are seeing patients with gastrointestinal disorders daily, in both inpatient, outpatient, and emergency department settings. This issue provides the physician assistant with the knowledge needed to evaluate and care for patients with these presentations.

This issue of *Physician Assistant Clinics*, with guest editor Jennifer Eames, provides an excellent review of several topics in gastroenterology. These articles will benefit the outpatient and inpatient surgical physician assistant. The articles can be divided into the upper and lower gastrointestinal tract. Esophageal disease is covered by Robinson, who discusses eosinophilic esophagitis, and Hastings, who covers refractory gastroesophageal reflux disease. Gastric disease is covered by Shell, who reviews the pathophysiology of peptic ulcer disease. Diseases of the liver are covered by Eames and Tran, who review hepatitis, and Bessette, who discusses nonalcoholic fatty liver disease. Intestinal disorders are covered by Martin, who reviews celiac disease, Butler, who covers colon cancer screening, Ladewski, who reviews irritable bowel syndrome, Miksa and Apperley, who discuss inflammatory bowel disease, and McDonald, who discusses acute gastrointestinal bleeding. Zahodnik provides an excellent review of evaluating patients for nutritional disorders.

Physician Assist Clin 6 (2021) xi–xii
https://doi.org/10.1016/j.cpha.2021.07.005
2405-7991/21/© 2021 Published by Elsevier Inc.

I hope you enjoy this issue. Our next issue will cover topics in Preventive Medicine.

James A. Van Rhee, MS, PA-C
Yale School of Medicine
Yale Physician Assistant Online Program
100 Church Street South, Suite A230
New Haven, CT 06519, USA

E-mail address:
james.vanrhee@yale.edu

Website:
http://www.paonline.yale.edu

REFERENCES

1. Santo L, Okeyode T. National ambulatory medical care survey: 2018 national summary tables. Available at: https://www.cdc.gov/nchs/data/ahcd/namcs_summary/2018-namcs-web-tables-508.pdf. Accessed August 2, 2021.
2. Peery AF, Crockett SD, Murphy CC, et al. Burden and cost of gastrointestinal, liver, and pancreatic diseases in the United States: update 2018. Gastroenterology 2019;156(1):254–72.e11. https://doi.org/10.1053/j.gastro.2018.08.063 [published correction appears in Gastroenterology 2019;156(6):1936].

Preface

Gastroenterology for Physician Assistants Today

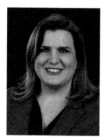

Jennifer R. Eames, MPAS, DHSc, PA-C
Editor

This *Physician Assistant Clinics* on Gastroenterology is an exciting work with clinical updates on many important topics, including esophageal, colonic, liver, and many other disorders. Gastroenterology (GI) is a too often overlooked specialty that can impact many areas of patients' daily lives. This issue includes updated guidelines for screening and treatment of common liver disorders, including nonalcoholic fatty liver disease and hepatitis C. Both disorders have increasing incidence and prevalence in the United States and will need primary care clinicians to be involved in the treatment for the epidemics to be curbed. Other sections include interesting discussions on upper GI disorders, like eosinophilic esophagitis, gastroesophageal reflux disease, and peptic ulcer disease. Irritable bowel syndrome and celiac disease management are discussed in detail, reviewing important concepts in patient management, and updating clinicians with best practices in helping patients with these complex disorders make positive progress in symptom control. In addition, the hot topic of nutritional deficiencies is updated with hard evidence for clinicians whose patients continue to ask about needs for the latest supplements and dietary trends. The work rounds out with lower GI topics, including inflammatory bowel disease and colon cancer screening recommendations.

It is the authors' and editing/publishing team's hope that these articles will help each reader take their GI knowledge to the next level and provide important updates to those in both clinical and educational settings. Each article was crafted with care by a practicing physician assistant (PA) or PA educator. This helps move the scholarly needle for the profession, modeling publishing as PA for the next generation. Please share these great works with others, cite them in writing and presentations, and use them as a base for building future articles.

It is the sincere hope of the publishing team, authors, and this editor that you find the works both approachable and informative. Each article contains "clinics care points"

https://doi.org/10.1016/j.cpha.2021.06.002
2405-7991/21/© 2021 Published by Elsevier Inc.
physicianassistant.theclinics.com

as a bulleted list that can serve as a quick reference for the topic pearls. In addition, figures have been added to attract reader interest and enhance the learning experience. While many find GI to be a complex, frustrating, or even less-palatable medical area of specialty, it has truly been a rewarding area of practice and lifelong love for this editor and many authors. That passion shines through this text and will bring readers both information and inspiration for better managing patients for the future.

Jennifer R. Eames, MPAS, DHSc, PA-C
Physician Assistant Department
Hardin-Simmons University
2200 Hickory
Box 16236
Abilene, TX 78698, USA

E-mail address:
jennifer.eames@hsutx.edu

Hepatitis C: Cure for a New Era

Jennifer R. Eames, MPAS, DHSc, PA-C[a],*, Bau Tran, MMS, PharmD, PA-C[b]

KEYWORDS

- Hepatitis C ● HCV ● Direct-acting antivirals ● Hepatocellular carcinoma

KEY POINTS

- Hepatitis C is a common and costly chronic viral infection globally and in the United States.
- New direct-acting antiviral medications can cure the infection and prevent future sequelae in less than 2 months with few side effects.
- Screening all adult patients for hepatitis C and treating it early can decrease global morbidity and mortality.

INTRODUCTION

It is estimated that approximately 170 million people are infected with the hepatitis C virus (HCV) globally.[1] This virus contributes to global morbidity and an estimated 1.3 million deaths across the globe each year.[2] Before the COVID-19 pandemic, hepatitis C was the most common blood-borne infection in the United-States, with an estimated 2.7 to 3.5 million active cases.[3] In 2010, this corresponded to an estimated 1.1% prevalence rate in noninstitutionalized adults in the United States.[4] Incidence of HCV is increasing this decade because of the worsening opioid epidemic, with most new infections in people younger than age 30.[5] Chronic hepatitis C was the most common cause of infection-related disease in the United States in 2016.[6] Most patients with the disease are asymptomatic and many are unaware of their diagnosis, making estimates of accurate numbers of infected individuals challenging.[3,4,7]

The World Health Organization (WHO) reports that 90% of infected people globally need to be identified and at least 80% treated to reach the goal of HCV eradication by 2030.[7,8] Many countries are setting agendas to address the public health crisis caused by HCV, and the Centers for Disease Control and Prevention (CDC), along with other US health authorities, have joined the fight increasingly in recent years.[7,9] The current number of health care specialists (gastroenterologists/hepatologists/infectious disease specialists) who provide most HCV therapy globally is insufficient to meet demand and need. For this reason, additional primary care clinicians need to become

[a] Department of Physician Assistant Studies, Hardin-Simmons University, 2200 Hickory Box 16236 Abilene, Texas 79698, USA; [b] UT Southwestern Department of Physician Assistant Studies, Texas Tech University College of Pharmacy, 5323 Harry Hines Blvd, Dallas TX 75390-9090, USA
* Corresponding author.
E-mail address: Jennifer.eames@hsutx.edu

Physician Assist Clin 6 (2021) 555–568
https://doi.org/10.1016/j.cpha.2021.05.002

more active in treating patients with HCV in the future to meet demand.[10-12] Physician assistants are commonly involved in treating HCV patients.[13] Primary care clinicians, including advance practice providers, have demonstrated safe and effective prescribing practices for HCV eradication using direct-acting antiviral drugs (DAAs) with efficacy rates similar to specialists.[11] New therapies have made a permanent cure of HCV in as few as 8 weeks of oral therapy and are urgently desired for use globally.[14]

BACKGROUND
History

HCV was identified as a virus in the year 1989.[1] HCV is a single-stranded RNA virus and has at least six known genotypes and many subtypes.[15] Although genotypes 1, 2, and 3 are most common in the United States, genotype 4 is most common in Egypt, genotype 5 is most common in Southern Africa, and genotype 6 is most common in Southeast Asia.[16] The virus has a high rate of mutation and can escape the host immune system even in the face of antibody formation in more than 75% of patients.[6] The HCV virus is a positive-strand RNA virus that causes inflammation of the liver.[17] Unlike other forms of hepatitis including hepatitis A virus (HAV) and hepatitis B virus (HBV), no vaccine currently exists for the HCV virus. Although HCV can cause acute, non-life-threatening illness, it most often results in an asymptomatic chronic infection.[7] For unknown reasons, many patients are able to clear the HCV infection without treatment; however, most patients develop chronic infection. Estimates for patients who clear the virus spontaneously range from 10% to 40%, with most others developing chronic disease.[17] Chronic infection is defined as the persistence of the virus for more than 6 months. Without treatment, approximately 20% to 30% of chronically infected patients develop cirrhosis over the upcoming 30 years.[10] As a lymphoproliferative virus, HCV is associated with several additional lymphoproliferative disorders including B-cell non-Hodgkin lymphoma.[18] By 2024, HCV is predicted to cost society $9.1 billion.[10] Achievement of a sustained virologic response (SVR) after treatment is associated with decreased risk of all-cause mortality and hepatocellular carcinoma (HCC).[17,19]

Risk Factors

Risk factors for infection with HCV include any activity that can transfer blood with virus from one human to another (**Table 1**). Commonly listed risk factors documented in the literature include injection drug use, incarceration, blood transfusion before 1992, hemodialysis, tattoos using unsanitary equipment, unprotected sexual contact, transmission at birth, having a history of HIV, nasal cocaine use, needlestick injuries,

Table 1	
Risk factors for contracting HCV[8,9,20,21]	
Injection drug use	Shared razors
Hemodialysis	Sexual contact
Unsterile tattoo practices	HIV
Vertical transmission	Exposure to blood products
Needlestick injury	Incarceration
Contaminated surgical instruments	Blood product transfusion before 1992
Nasal cocaine use	Solid organ transplant

exposure to blood products, and surgical procedures using unsterilized instruments.[8,9,20,21] It is known that the HCV virus can exist on surfaces for greater than 24 hours, making use of nonsterilized items for medical procedures or items involved in the injection of drugs (eg, cotton, cookers) possible sources of infection. Even vats of tattoo ink when not changed between clients has been hypothesized as a potential source of HCV spread.

Epidemiology

The estimated rates of chronic hepatitis C are higher in non-Hispanic Black patients than in non-Hispanic White patients in the United States.[4] Additionally, indigenous peoples are disproportionately impacted by HCV burden.[4,22] It is estimated that more than two-thirds of those currently infected were born between 1945 and 1965 as part of the "Baby Boomer" generation.[3,4] Although most cases of HCV infection are found in adults of the Baby Boomer generation, recent increases in HCV incidence are related largely to younger people who inject drugs.[19]

Disease Complications

HCV infection is a leading cause of liver transplants and the cause of more than half of primary liver cancers.[7] HCC is the most common primary liver cancer and the fastest-rising cause of death from cancer in America.[18] Delayed HCV treatment can lead to cirrhosis, which increases a patient's risk for HCC and, in rare cases, intrahepatic cholangiocarcinoma.[18] Previously populations who abused alcohol or intravenous drugs were not often granted therapy options by providers or insurers until abstinent from all substances for a period of 6 to 12 months at minimum. However, new evidence argues against this requirement of abstinence from substances and argues in favor of early treatment despite substance abuse for public health and individual improved outcomes.[18] Infection with HCV is also associated with the development of mixed cryoglobulinemia, lichen planus of the skin, B-cell non-Hodgkin lymphoma, and many autoimmune disorders.[1]

PATIENT EVALUATION
Screening

It is currently recommended to screen all persons 18 to 79 years of age at least once and screen pregnant women with each pregnancy (**Fig. 1**).[9,23] Repeat screening is recommended for those with risk factors. Universal screening strategies have been found to be cost-effective from a public health standpoint in the era of highly effective, pangenotypic, rapidly effective DAAs with few side effects.[7] Before the CDC recommendation changes in 2012 and US Preventive Services Task Force (USPSTF) recommendation expansion again in 2020, it was estimated that less than 2% of Baby Boomers had been screened for HCV by their health care provider.[3,23] Baby Boomers have increased risk because of possible exposure earlier in life through various means (eg, unsterilized medical tools, transfusions, intravenous drug use experimentation).[6] The updated CDC and USPSTF recommendations for widespread screening have been effective with screening rates cumulatively increasing from 16% in 2012 to 82% in 2017.[20] It is hoped that the CDC's latest recommendations to screen all adults will improve these rates even more in future years.

HCV screening gaps may be related to a lack of patient access to care.[3] These gaps are more apparent in minority groups and rural populations. One study of veteran populations noted a significant increase in screening after the first CDC recommendation for a one-time screening of all Baby Boomers.[3] The recommended screening test is an

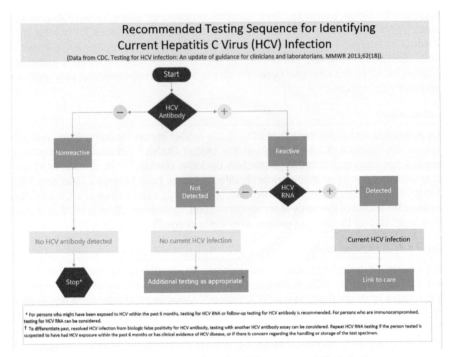

Fig. 1. Recommended testing sequence for identifying current HCV infection.

HCV antibody test with reflex HCV RNA polymerase chain reaction (PCR) testing.[21] It is estimated that up to 26% of patients with acute HCV spontaneously clear the infection within 6 months of exposure and will not have active disease at the time of diagnosis as detectable by the reflex HCV RNA PCR testing.[4] This would mean that these individuals would have a positive antibody test but a negative HCV RNA PCR test.

Testing for the HCV-antibody is done from serum samples or buccal swabs.[6] Positive HCV antibody can indicate active or past infection with the HCV virus.[21] There is no need to repeat HCV antibody testing in a known positive patient because once positive, it remains positive. One study found that between 2006 and 2010 inappropriate repeat antibody screening cost New York City approximately $14 million.[20] Although a positive HCV antibody is durable, HCV RNA PCR levels can fluctuate and become undetectable after treatment; therefore, testing is recommended before and after therapy.

Before Starting Therapy (Treatment Naive)

Initial visits
When evaluating a patient with a diagnosis of hepatitis C, a thorough history must be done to assess potential risk factors and a history of any prior treatment attempts.[24] Additionally, the initial visits are an excellent time to engage in patient education on ways to avoid spreading the disease to others. Work-up of a patient with established chronic HCV infection includes evaluation of liver function tests through markers including alanine aminotransferase, aspartate aminotransferase, alkaline phosphatase, and γ-glutamyltransferase (**Table 2**).[6] However, most patients exhibit normal liver enzymes and even those with advanced fibrosis could exhibit normal

Table 2 Initial laboratory studies[6]	
Stage hepatic fibrosis	Hepatic function panel
Assess possible medication interactions	eGFR
Patient education on therapy (side effects, adherence)	Quantitative HCV RNA (viral load)
CBC	Hepatitis B virus testing
INR	HIV testing
	Child-Turcotte-Pugh score
	Pregnancy testing and counseling

Abbreviations: CBC, complete blood count; eGFR, estimated glomerular filtration rate; INR, international normalized ratio.

transaminases in up to 40% of cases.[6] Measurement of total platelet counts, albumin, bilirubin, and prothrombin time can also help to indicate if liver fibrosis is present.[6] Unfortunately, lack of insurance coverage and access to care for these evaluations is a barrier to treatment with 29.6% of HCV-infected patients being uninsured in the United States.[25]

HIV and HCV have overlapping risk factors and potential treatment complications can occur in patients infected with both viruses; for this reason, HIV screening should be done on all patients with HCV.[6,21] HBV screening is also recommended before treatment, followed by immunization for HBV if no active disease is present.[21]

Liver biopsy was previously recommended for all patients to stage fibrosis but is no longer considered standard of care or fundamental to the evaluation of patients with chronic HCV in the era of new DAAs.[21] However, it is recommended that the clinician establish the patient's diagnosis of cirrhosis before new therapy initiation because different drugs have duration differences for patients with cirrhosis versus patients without cirrhosis.[6,21] One of the most reliable and accurate noninvasive measures of liver fibrosis in patients with chronic kidney disease (CKD) is the aminotransferase-to-platelet ratio index (APRI).[6] This ratio is calculated as [(aspartate aminotransferase level/upper limit of normal)/platelets] $\times$ 100 and online calculators exist for clinicians. The APRI score has a traditional two-sided cutoff to predict fibrosis of the liver of F3 or greater less than 0.4 predicting no likely significant fibrosis and greater than 2 predicting cirrhosis.[26]

Often, APRI is used in combination with another score, such as Fibrosis-4 or FibroTest for enhanced accuracy.[27] Alternately, direct imaging through traditional techniques, such as ultrasound or elastography techniques, for assessment of liver fibrosis is helpful when evaluating a patient for evidence of cirrhosis.

Although most patients are asymptomatic, extrahepatic manifestations of HCV can occur in multiple organ systems including complications with the kidneys, skin, central nervous system, cardiovascular system, immune system, and endocrine system.[6] HCV remains a leading cause of needed liver transplants in the United States and globally.[5] Historically, those most likely to receive treatment quickly were those with Medicare and/or private insurance and those with more severe disease.[27] This needs to change if the goal of universal treatment and eradication of HCV by 2030 is to be achieved globally.

Note that the presence of an HCV antibody does not confer immunity as other types of hepatitis antibodies (eg, HAV or HBV).[6] Specifically, once a patient is treated and/or has their HCV resolve spontaneously as evidenced by no active measurable circulating virus and the presence of persistent antibody, they can potentially become reinfected later. The primary goal of HCV therapy is to achieve an SVR and thereby prevent worsening liver fibrosis and end-stage complications.[28] After DAA therapy, laboratory monitoring includes a measurement of HCV RNA by PCR 12 weeks after therapy completion to check for SVR.[19]

Hepatocellular carcinoma screening

Mortality for HCC is increasing faster than other cancers.[12] Only 20% of patients have a survival rate greater than 5 years after the diagnosis of HCC.[12] Patients with HCV should be screened for HCC because HCV infection and cirrhosis are known risk factors for HCC. This screening should occur initially with imaging when possible and serum α-fetoprotein level tumor marker every 6 months.[6] The most common imaging modality is ultrasound.

SPECIAL POPULATIONS
Use of Injection Drugs

People who inject drugs are the top population at risk for new HCV infections in the United States yet are treated at less than a 15% rate by some providers.[13,22] Sadly, there is poor recognition that HCV is a curable disease by patients with a history of injection drug use with less than 50% aware of available curative therapy.[25] Many providers are reluctant to treat patients actively using street drugs for fear of loss to follow-up and reinfection concerns.[13] Historically, some insurers have even rejected treatment coverage for those with substance use disorders.[22] However, evidence exists that HCV treatment is linked with better outcomes for patients to later overcome addictions.[13] New oral treatments are able to be effective so quickly that the cost has been shown to be outweighed by the benefits even in people who actively inject drugs.[13] More than 6 years ago, one of the largest health care providers in the nation, the Veterans Affairs health care program, recommended the removal of the minimum abstinence time before HCV treatment.[18] Furthermore, the American Association for the Study of Liver Diseases (AASLD), WHO, and Infectious Disease Society of America all have documented their support for prioritizing HCV therapy for people who inject drugs and people with alcohol use disorders.[18]

Renal Impairment

Hepatitis C infection is common in patients with CKD and history of hemodialysis with a prevalence rate of 10% to 16% worldwide.[1,6] Patients with CKD are approximately five times more likely than the general population to have HCV.[6] This increased risk may be related to the history of blood transfusions in many CKD patients before blood screening began in the early 1990s.[1,6] Studies show reduced life expectancy for HCV-positive transplant recipients of approximately 10 years.[6] For this reason, patients with HCV awaiting transplant are now encouraged to undergo therapy with DAAs before transplant if possible, to avoid interactions with post-transplant immunosuppressive drugs.[1] Nonsofosbuvir-based regimens are preferred for patients with stage 4 and 5 CKD because of possible renal impact.[6] Timing of medications for patients on and off dialysis becomes particularly important with patients with CKD because dialysis can impact absorption and timing of drug absorption is impacted by renal function impairment or other drug interactions.[14]

The new, safer HCV therapies have opened a new donor pool for kidney and other solid-organ donors. Now, patients are increasingly willing to accept an organ transplant from a patient with known HCV infection because of the high cure rates of HCV with new DAA regimens taken by the organ recipient post-transplant.[29] In patients considering receiving an organ transplant from an HCV-infected donor, informed consent, insurance review of covered DAAs, and ongoing surveillance are critical for success.[29]

HIV Coinfection

Reports estimate that between 5% and 30% of people living with HIV are also infected with HCV.[24] There are geographic variations of HIV/HCV coinfection that have some basis in risk-related factors. Because HIV/HCV coinfection is known to accelerate liver fibrosis, patients with both infections are especially important to treat whenever possible. HCV coinfected patients experience a longer wait time to treatment initiation than monoinfected patients.[24] However, with consistent use of the new DAAs, rates of SVR in HIV/HCV coinfected patients are similar to rates in monoinfected patients with HCV alone.[24,30] Some state Medicaid payors and other private payors limit access to DAAs based on costs, but the value of dual treatment over a lifetime has been demonstrated.[30] However, the potential exists for drug-drug interactions with HIV and HCV therapies; thus, caution must be used when prescribing. For this reason, coordination between treating providers for DAAs and **highly active antiretroviral therapy** is critical for patient best outcomes.[24,30] With high-level collaboration and provider coordination, one study demonstrated no difference in drug-drug interactions between HIV/HCV coinfected patients and monoinfected patients.[24,30] Patient quality of life in those living with HIV has increased after achieving SVR from HCV.[30]

Pregnancy and Children

Vertical transmission is the leading risk factor for pediatric HCV infections globally and studies of treatment in pregnant patients living with chronic HCV infection are ongoing.[2] As stated, the CDC, AASLD, and USPSTF all support screening mothers for HCV with each pregnancy.[9,21,23] Older therapies that included ribavirin, a known teratogen, excluded pregnant patients from treatment of any kind; however, this is no longer the case in the new era of DAAs. Although animal studies show that DAAs are metabolized differently during pregnancy and likely cross the placental barrier and into breast milk, a recent meta-analysis shows that they are likely safe later in pregnancy, typically in the early third trimester.[2] Risk reduction for vertical transmission has been documented by performing C-sections instead of vaginal births and eliminating the use of scalp intrauterine fetal monitors during labor.[2] Currently, the literature lacks large-scale data related to the safety and efficacy of DAAs in pregnancy, so more studies are needed and encouraged.[2] Testing for HCV antibodies is not reliable in children until after 18 months of age. Pediatric treatment with DAAs for older children (>12 years) was approved by the Food and Drug Administration in 2017.[2]

Hepatitis B Coinfection

Patients infected with HCV have HBV exposure rates at six times the rate of HCV-negative patients.[31] Such high rates may be related to overlapping risk factors for contracting the viruses. Having both infections puts patients at a significantly increased risk for cirrhosis and HCC.[31] Although both viruses can be treated in patients simultaneously, it is recommended that coinfected patients be managed by specialists outside of primary care.[6] The treatment of HBV is beyond the scope of this discussion. However, the literature supports encouraging all HCV-positive patients to be vaccinated for HAV and HBV if not actively infected even though the rate of HBV vaccine nonresponse is high in patients with HCV.[31]

THERAPEUTIC OPTIONS
Historical Treatment

The discovery of HCV, previously termed non-A, non-B hepatitis, in 1989 allowed for advanced research to unravel the critical components of the devastating virus that has affected many around the world. Houghton[32] in the 1980s replicated and sequenced the genome of HCV that paved the way for the current pharmacologic management. In the early 1990s, pharmacologic treatment consisted of a course of non-PEGylated interferon alpha-2a or alpha-2b monotherapy for 24 or 48 weeks, depending on the genotype.[33] This regimen required injections three times per week and was associated with significant side effects including nausea/vomiting, headaches, chills, depression, suicidal ideation, neutropenia, thrombocytopenia, autoimmune disease, and liver damage.[34] Success in clearing the virus with this regimen was less than or equal to 10% and resulted in poor outcomes. Ribavirin was added to the regimen to increase the SVR rate. This resulted in improved outcomes and SVR rates of approximately 30% to 40%. Although this dual therapy had improved SVR rates, the improvement was heavily reliant on the genotype with lower cure rates for genotype 1 and 4. Unfortunately, despite improved SVR, ribavirin added additional side effects of anemia, respiratory complications, and teratogenicity to this dual therapy often preventing patients from completing their treatment course.[35]

With the advent of a PEGylated formulation of interferon-alfa 2a and 2b toward the end of 1990s, this new formulation altered the pharmacokinetic properties of the medication allowing for once weekly injection with better absorption, reduced distribution, and decreased elimination. This ultimately improved the rate of inhibition of viral replication and increased SVR rates.[35] A 24- to 48-week course of this regimen boosted the SVR rates for genotype 2, 3, 5, and 6 to 80%; however, patients with genotype 1 had a much lower success rate of around 40%.[33]

Although some patients could be cured, this regimen was associated with substantial toxicity and many patients were not candidates for therapy because of nonsofosbuvir contraindications to interferon or ribavirin. Major contraindications to the use of interferon are uncontrolled depression or psychosis (neuropsychiatric effects; unknown), autoimmune disease (immune-modulatory effects), and decompensated liver disease (hepatocyte necrosis and necroinflammatory effects). The side effects and contraindications combined with poor outcomes (especially in genotype 1 and 4 infections) prompted the need for newer, more efficacious and less toxic treatment modalities.[33]

Current Treatment

Advances in gene mapping technology with the discovery of target sites of action allowed for the development of new DAAs to treat HCV more effectively.[1] Proteolytic enzymes modify the virus's polyproteins into four structural and six nonstructural (NS) proteins. The NS proteins that are targeted by current therapies are the NS3/4A, NS5A, and NS5B proteins and are responsible for cleaving polyproteins into their respective structural and NS proteins, mediating interferon resistance, and RNA-dependent RNA polymerase activity, respectively.

Treatment today has changed dramatically because of groundbreaking discoveries that have significantly improved cure rates to greater than 95% across all genotypes with fewer, less severe side effects and withdrawal, leading to reduced patient morbidity and mortality.[19] Treatments, including DAAs, are tailored to target multiple genotypes with a specified treatment duration. To date, the newest agents developed and marketed as combination products since 2015 have the highest safety and

Table 3

Commonly available direct-acting antivirals and site of action[34]

NS3/4A Inhibitors	NS5A Inhibitor	NS5B Inhibitors
Glecaprevir	Daclatasvir	Sofosbuvir
Grazoprevir	Elbasvir	Dasabuvir
Paritaprevir	Ledipasvir	
Simeprevir	Ombitasvir	
Voxilaprevir	Pibrentasvir	
	Velpatasvir	

Source: Lexi-Drugs. Lexicomp. Wolters Kluwer Health, Inc. Riverwoods, IL. Available at: http://online.lexi.com. Accessed November 5, 2020.

efficacy with a significantly lower dropout rate than regimens previously established containing interferon.[27] Patients who completed DAA therapy had improved quality of life scores 12 weeks after completing therapy.[19] In contrast to the old 48-week regimen, the cure rates of the new 8- to 12-week regimens are consistently greater than 95% to 99% in some populations providing hope for a potential worldwide eradication of this disease.[10] A list of current therapy is provided in **Table 3**.

Specific studies reviewing the safety and efficacy of treatments with each different genotype have been reviewed in the literature and DAAs approved for use currently have cure rates that exceed 95% for most patients.[36] Given all of this information, the AASLD now recommends treating all patients actively infected with HCV without a limited lifespan.[21,27] The AASLD and Infectious Diseases Society of America provide simplified initial HCV treatment guidelines for treatment-naive adults without cirrhosis and those with compensated cirrhosis. This information is accessible at https://www.hcvguidelines.org/treatment-naive. Initial recommended regimens are glecaprevir/

Table 4

Top two treatments for HCV[a] in treatment-naive patients

Drug	Epclusa (sofosbuvir – NS5B inhibitor/velpatasvir – NS5A inhibitor)	Mavyret (glecaprevir – NS3/4A inhibitor/pibrentasvir – NS5A inhibitor)
Indications	Genotype 1–6 infection	Genotype 1–6 infection with or without compensated cirrhosis
Dosing	400/100 mg once daily × 12 wk	100/40 mg: 3 tablets once daily with food × 8 wk (without cirrhosis) or × 12 wk (with compensated cirrhosis)
Renal adjustment	No dosage adjustment necessary	No dosage adjustment necessary
Hepatic adjustment	No dosage adjustment necessary	Mild impairment (Child-Pugh class A): no dosage adjustment necessary Moderate to severe impairment (Child-Pugh class B or C): use is contraindicated
Adverse effects	Fatigue, headache, irritability	Nausea, fatigue, headache, pruritus, diarrhea

[a] Lexicomp. Wolters Kluwer Health, Inc. Riverwoods, IL. Available at: http://online.lexi.com. Accessed November 5, 2020.

Table 5
Common drug-drug interactions with DAAs

Concomitant Medications	Velpatasvir/Sofosbuvir	Glecaprevir/Pibrentasvir
Acid-reducing agents	Antacids H2RA PPI	H2RA PPI
Antiarrhythmics	Amiodarone Dronedarone Digoxin Quinidine	Amiodarone Dronedarone Quinidine
Anticoagulant and antiplatelet agents	Apixaban Dabigatran Edoxaban Rivaroxaban Ticagrelor Warfarin	Dabigatran Apixaban Edoxaban Rivaroxaban Ticagrelor Warfarin
Anticonvulsants and barbiturates	Amobarbital Carbamazepine Eslicarbazepine Oxcarbazepine Phenobarbital Phenytoin Primidone Rufinamide	Amobarbital Carbamazepine Eslicarbazepine Oxcarbazepine Phenobarbital Phenytoin Primidone Rufinamide
Antihypertensive	Diltiazem	Aliskiren Enalapril Eplerenone Irbesartan Isradipine Non-DHP CCB Olmesartan Telmisartan
Antipsychotics, 2nd generation		Aripiprazole Clozapine Paliperidone Quetiapine
Antiretrovirals	http://www.hcvguidelines.org/unique-populations/hiv-hcv	
Azole antifungals		Ketoconazole Posaconazole
Cholesterol-lowering agents	Atorvastatin Fluvastatin Lovastatin Pitavastatin Rosuvastatin Simvastatin	Atorvastatin Lovastatin Simvastatin Ezetimibe Fluvastatin Gemfibrozil Pitavastatin Pravastatin Rosuvastatin
Glucocorticoids		Dexamethasone
Heart failure agents	Bosentan	Bosentan Ambrisentan

(continued on next page)

Table 5 (continued)		
Concomitant Medications	**Velpatasvir/Sofosbuvir**	**Glecaprevir/Pibrentasvir**
Herbals	St. John's wort	St. John's wort
Loop diuretics		
Macrolide antimicrobials		Erythromycin Telithromycin
Phosphodiesterase-5 inhibitors		
Rifamycin antimicrobials	Rifabutin Rifampicin Rifapentine	Rifabutin Rifampicin Rifapentine Rifaximin

Abbreviations: DHP CCB, dihydropyridine calcium channel blocker; H2RA, histamine H_2 antagonist; non-DHP CCB, nondihydropyridine calcium channel blocker; PPI, proton pump inhibitor.

Green indicates coadministration is safe, yellow indicates a dose change or additional monitoring is warranted, and red indicates the combination should be avoided. Specific concomitant medications or medication classes with actual or theoretic potential for interaction are listed in the box.

Data from CDC. CDC.gov. https://www.cdc.gov/hepatitis/hcv/management.htm.

pibrentasvir (Mavyret) and sofosbuvir/velpatasvir (Epclusa) for 8 weeks and 12 weeks, respectively.[21] The primary goal of HCV therapy is to achieve an SVR and thereby prevent worsening liver fibrosis and end-stage complications.[28] Although there are other available treatment options, the agents listed previously are reviewed here.

Some therapies have recommendations about how best to take them (with or without food) and recommendations for storage (ie, <30°C).[37] A common and often overlooked drug-drug interaction involves DAAs and some proton pump inhibitors.[16] Patients should be counseled regarding over-the-counter and prescription medications (eg, proton pump inhibitors) to avoid while on certain therapies. Rarely, cutaneous rashes have been noted in patients taking sofosbuvir; however, these were typically mild.[38] In addition, patients being treated with amiodarone should not receive sofosbuvir-based regimens because of risk of life-threatening arrhythmias. Because of its long half-life, it is advised that persons should be off amiodarone for at least 6 months before initiating sofosbuvir. If the decision is made to start sofosbuvir in this setting, continued vigilance for bradycardia should be exercised.[37] Counseling and education by prescribing providers and pharmacists before the start of DAA therapy are essential to patient success and avoiding drug-drug interactions, and unexpected adverse events by patients.[24] Furthermore, laboratory monitoring after DAA therapy includes a measurement of HCV RNA by PCR 12 weeks after therapy completion to check for SVR12. **Table 4** summarizes the top two treatments for HCV in treatment-naive patients focusing on indications based on genotype, dosing, renal and hepatic adjustments when applicable, and common adverse effects. Commonly encountered drug interactions with DAAs are listed in **Table 5**.

SUMMARY

Unlike other viruses, HCV is now a truly curable disease.[17] Although cost continues to be a barrier for universal treatment in the United States and globally, data show that the cost/benefit ratio makes the use of DAAs worthwhile in many countries worldwide. This trend of affordability could continue to improve as governments negotiate with pharmaceutical companies.[39] Additionally, companies around the world are working to develop lower-cost DAAs for the market and studies are ongoing for new therapies. Discussions about flexibilities under the World Trade Organization's agreement about international intellectual property rights will play an important role in the future of HCV drug costs.[15,39] Although historically, primary care providers reported limited knowledge of and experience with hepatitis C treatment, that trend is changing in the new era of DAA use.[25] Using new DAA agents, with collaboration and coordination among all clinicians, the WHO's goal of eradication of HCV globally is truly within reach.

CLINICS CARE POINTS

- All adults should be screened for HCV regardless of risk factors (CDC).
- Two new therapies for HCV provide cure for more than 95% of patients in less than 3 months.
- Most patients without cirrhosis who have never been treated before are cured in 8 weeks.
- Every patient with HCV should be screened for cirrhosis, HBV, and HIV before treatment.
- HCV patients with cirrhosis should be evaluated for HCC every 6 months.
- On HCV treatment, no serial laboratory monitoring is recommended for most patients.
- Because of ease of oral therapy, primary care clinicians, including physician assistants, can manage HCV treatment.
- Pharmacists and clinicians should work together during HCV treatment to avoid drug-drug interactions.

DISCLOSURE STATEMENT

The authors have nothing to disclose.

REFERENCES

1. Pagan J, Ladino M, Roth D. Treating hepatitis C virus in dialysis patients: how, when, and why? Semin Dial 2018;32(2):152–8.
2. Freriksen J, van Seyen M, Judd A, et al. Review article: direct-acting antivirals for the treatment of HCV during pregnancy and lactation - implications for maternal dosing, foetal exposure, and safety for mother and child. Aliment Pharmacol Ther 2019;50(7):738–50.
3. Manjelievskaia J, Brown D, Shriver C, et al. CDC screening recommendation for baby boomers and hepatitis C virus testing in the US Military health system. Public Health Rep 2017;132(5):579–84.
4. Hall E, Rosenberg E, Sullivan P. Estimates of state-level chronic hepatitis C virus infection, stratified by race and sex, United States, 2010. BMC Infect Dis 2018; 18(1). https://doi.org/10.1186/s12879-018-3133-6.
5. Chhatwal J, Sussman N. Universal Screening for hepatitis C: an important step in virus elimination. Clin Gastroenterol Hepatol 2019;17(5):835–7.
6. Cottone C, Bhamidimarri K. Evaluating CKD/ESRD patient with hepatitis C infection: how to interpret diagnostic testing and assess liver injury. Semin Dial 2019; 32(2):119–26.
7. Cortesi P, Barca R, Giudicatti G, et al. Systematic review: economic evaluations of HCV screening in the direct-acting antivirals era. Aliment Pharmacol Ther 2019; 49(9):1126–33.

8. World Health Organization. Hepat C. 2020. Who.int. Available at: https://www.who.int/news-room/fact-sheets/detail/hepatitis-c. Accessed October 5, 2020.

9. Centers for Disease Control & Prevention. Recommendations for prevention and control of hepatitis C virus (HCV) infection and HCV-related chronic disease | HCV | Division of Viral Hepatitis | CDC. 2020. Cdc.gov. Available at: https://www.cdc.gov/hepatitis/hcv/management.htm. Accessed October 6, 2020.

10. Zullig L, Bhatia H, Gellad Z, et al. Adoption of direct-acting antiviral medications for hepatitis C: a retrospective observational study. BMC Health Serv Res 2019;19(1). https://doi.org/10.1186/s12913-019-4349-x.

11. Kattakuzhy S, Gross C, Emmanuel B, et al. Expansion of treatment for hepatitis C virus infection by task shifting to community-based nonspecialist providers. Ann Intern Med 2017;167(5):311.

12. Tenner L, Melhado T, Bobadilla R, et al. The cost of cure: barriers to access for hepatitis C virus treatment in South Texas. J Oncol Pract 2019;15(2):61–3.

13. Asher A, Portillo C, Cooper B, et al. Clinicians' views of hepatitis C virus treatment candidacy with direct-acting antiviral regimens for people who inject drugs. Subst Use Misuse 2016;51(9):1218–23.

14. Cohen E, Liapakis A. Pharmacokinetics and important drug-drug interactions to remember when treating advanced chronic kidney disease patients with hepatitis C direct acting anti-viral therapy. Semin Dial 2018;32(2):141–51.

15. Abo-Talib N, El-Ghobashy M, Tammam M. Spectrophotometric Methods for Simultaneous Determination of Sofosbuvir and Ledipasvir (HARVONI Tablet): comparative study with two generic products. J AOAC Int 2017;100(4):976–84.

16. Miller M. Sofosbuvir–velpatasvir: a single-tablet treatment for hepatitis C infection of all genotypes. Am J Health-System Pharm 2017;74(14):1045–52.

17. Zhang X. Direct anti-HCV agents. Acta Pharmaceutica Sinica B 2016;6(1):26–31.

18. Barua S, Sprecht-Walsch S, Weiss Z, et al. Intrahepatic cholangiocarcinoma in a patient with hepatitis C: a cautionary tale. R Med J 2020;30–4.

19. Chou R, Dana T, Fu R, et al. Screening for hepatitis C virus infection in adolescents and adults. JAMA 2020;323(10):976.

20. Coppock D, Chou E, Gracely E, et al. Hepatitis C antibody screening and determinants of initial and duplicate screening in the baby boomer patients of six urban primary care clinics. PLoS One 2020;15(7):e0235778.

21. AASLD-IDSA. Recommendations for testing, managing, and treating hepatitis C | HCV Guidance. 2020. Hcvguidelines.org. Available at: https://www.hcvguidelines.org/. Accessed November 5, 2020.

22. Page K, Cox A, Lum P. Opioids, hepatitis C virus infection, and the missing vaccine. Am J Public Health 2018;108(2):156–7.

23. USPSTF. Updated hepatitis C screening recommendation. 2020. HHS.gov. Available at: https://www.hhs.gov/hepatitis/blog/2020/03/04/uspstf-issues-updated-hepatitis-c-screening-recommendation.html. Accessed November 5, 2020.

24. Zuckerman A, Douglas A, Whelchel K, et al. Pharmacologic management of HCV treatment in patients with HCV monoinfection vs. HIV/HCV coinfection: does co-infection really matter? PLoS One 2019;14(11):e0225434.

25. McGowan C, Fried M. Barriers to hepatitis C treatment. Liver Int 2011;32:151–6.

26. Lin ZH, Xin YN, Dong QJ, et al. Performance of the aspartate aminotransferase-to-platelet ratio index for the staging of hepatitis C-related fibrosis: an updated meta-analysis. Hepatology 2011;53:726–36.

27. Kwo P, Puenpatom A, Zhang Z, et al. Initial uptake, time to treatment, and real-world effectiveness of all-oral direct-acting antivirals for hepatitis C virus infection

in the United States: a retrospective cohort analysis. PLoS One 2019;14(8): e0218759.

28. Sarfraz M, Rabbani A, Shahzad Manzoor M, et al. Virological responses of velpatasvir/sofosbuvir in patients with HCV genotype 3. J Univ Med Dental Coll 2020; 11(1):9–14.

29. Karpel H, Ali N, Lawson N, et al. Successful A2 to B deceased donor kidney transplant after desensitization for high-strength non-HLA antibody made possible by utilizing a hepatitis C positive donor. Case Rep Transpl 2020; 2020:1–6.

30. Patel S, Jayaweera D, Althoff K, et al. Real-world efficacy of direct acting antiviral therapies in patients with HIV/HCV. PLoS One 2020;15(2):e0228847.

31. Ashhab A, Rodin H, Campos M, et al. Response to hepatitis B virus vaccination in individuals with chronic hepatitis C virus infection. PLoS One 2020;15(8): e0237398.

32. Houghton M. Discovery of the hepatitis C virus. Liver Int 2009;29(SUPPL. 1):82–8.

33. Burstow N, Mohamed Z, Gomaa A, et al. Hepatitis C treatment: where are we now? Int J Gen Med 2017;10:39–52.

34. Lexi-Drugs. Lexicomp. Wolters Kluwer Health, Inc. Riverwoods, IL. Available at: http://online.lexi.com. Accessed November 5, 2020.

35. Dahiya M, Hussaini T, Yoshida E. The revolutionary changes in hepatitis c treatment: a concise review. Br Columbia Med J 2019;61(2):72–7.

36. Due O, Chaikledkaew U, Genuino A, et al. Systematic review with meta-analysis: efficacy and safety of direct-acting antivirals for chronic hepatitis C genotypes 5 and 6. Biomed Res Int 2019;2019:1–12.

37. Traynor K. Oral therapy approved for chronic HCV infection of all genotypes. Am J Health-System Pharm 2016;73(15):1120.

38. Macklis P, Dulmage B, Evans B, et al. Cutaneous adverse events in newly approved FDA non-cancer drugs: a systematic review. Drugs R D 2020;20(3): 171–87.

39. Chen G, Wei L, Chen J, et al. Will sofosbuvir/ledipasvir (Harvoni) be cost-effective and affordable for Chinese patients infected with hepatitis C virus? An economic analysis using real-world data. PLoS One 2016;11(6):e0155934.

Review of Celiac Disease
Clinical Manifestations, Diagnosis, and Management

Helen Martin, DHSC, PA-C, DFAAPA

KEYWORDS

- Celiac disease • Malabsorption • Nontropical sprue • Wheat allergy
- Gluten sensitivity enteropathy • Gluten-free diet • Celiac spruce • Genetic screening

KEY POINTS

- Typical symptoms include weight loss, diarrhea, abdominal distention, iron deficiency, and osteoporosis.
- Positive result of small bowel biopsy.
- Positive serologic marker result.
- Clinical improvement with a gluten-free diet.

INTRODUCTION

Celiac disease is a chronic, small intestinal immune-mediated enteropathy initiated by exposure to dietary gluten in genetically predisposed individuals. This disease is characterized by specific autoantibodies against tissue transglutaminase 2 (anti-tTG2), endomysium, and/or deamidated gliadin peptide (DGP).[1]

Celiac disease is a lifelong condition that damages the lining of the small intestines and prevents it from absorbing parts of food that are important for proper health. The clinical presentation of celiac disease was first described in 1888, by Dr Samuel Gee who published the first complete modern description of the clinical picture of celiac disease and theorized on the importance of diet in its control. The cause of celiac disease was eventually discovered to be an autoimmune reaction to gliadin, a gluten protein found in wheat plus secalin in rye and hordien in barley. The lining of the small bowel is flattened, which interferes with the absorption of nutrients.[2] Disease presentation varies from one patient to the next, but the cause has remained constant. Because of the variety of symptoms patients display, it became known as the "great masquerader" and oftentimes took many years to accurately diagnose.

2811 Stonestown Drive, Charleston, SC 29414, USA
E-mail address: marthele@musc.edu

Physician Assist Clin 6 (2021) 569–580
https://doi.org/10.1016/j.cpha.2021.06.001
2405-7991/21/© 2021 Elsevier Inc. All rights reserved.

Celiac disease presents differently in each person. Celiac disease can present with many symptoms, including typical gastrointestinal symptoms (eg, diarrhea, steatorrhea, weight loss, bloating, flatulence, abdominal pain) and also nongastrointestinal abnormalities (eg, abnormal liver function tests, iron deficiency anemia, bone disease, skin disorders, and many other protean manifestations).[3] One patient may exhibit diarrhea, whereas another may experience constipation or abdominal pain. Some patient may be depressed or irritable, whereas others have no symptoms at all.[4]

The average time for a symptomatic person to be diagnosed is 11 years. This time increases an individual's risk of developing autoimmune disorders, neurologic problems, osteoporosis, and even cancer.[4] Many individuals with celiac disease have additional autoimmune diseases such as type 1 diabetes, rheumatoid arthritis, autoimmune thyroid or liver disease, Addison disease or Sjögren syndrome, Down syndrome, or Turner syndrome. If 1 member of a patient's family has it, about 1 of 10 other family members likely has it. Oftentimes, some individuals do not even know they have it. These individuals may have this disease without getting sick. In life, something triggers or activates the disease, and this could be severe stress, physical injury, infection, childbirth, or surgery.[5] Factors that may predispose someone to celiac disease are type 1 diabetes, Down syndrome, and thyroid disease.

The prevalence of celiac disease has been estimated as high as approximately 0.5% to 1% of the general population with a female predominance.[6]

DEFINITIONS: TYPES OF CELIAC DISEASE

The spectrum of celiac disease can present in many different forms.

- Typical (classical) (gastrointestinal symptoms): patients present with malabsorption disorders (diarrhea, steatorrhea, weight loss, and nutritional deficiencies and growth failure).[7]
- Atypical (extraintestinal symptoms): anemia, infertility, fatigue, and bloating.[7]
- Latent: no intestinal damage despite ingesting gluten but later develops villous change.[7]
- Silent: (asymptomatic but discovered via routine screening) has a positive serology test result but no symptoms or signs of celiac disease.[7]
- Potential: normal biopsy result but negative serology result.[7]
- Nonresponsive and refractory celiac disease: continuous and/or persistent symptoms, elevated antibodies or small intestinal damage even after following a strict gluten-free diet.[7]

BACKGROUND

Celiac disease damages the lining of the small intestines and prevents the proper absorption of food, which leads to other health conditions.

Gluten has to be present in food in order for the body to recognize and react to it. Gluten-free diet is the only treatment of this common genetic autoimmune condition. People have to eat food that contains gluten to manifest celiac disease.[8] Symptoms generally improve for most people with celiac disease who stick to a gluten-free diet.[9] Celiac disease occurs in people of all ages and ethnicities but seems to be most common in Caucasians of northern European descent. More than 95% of affected patients have HLA-DQ2 and/or HLA-DQ8 mutations. Celiac disease is found in approximately 1:22 of individuals with affected first-degree family members.[10]

Although the historical clinical presentation of celiac disease seemed to be in children, now celiac disease is most often diagnosed in individuals in their *50s* and *60s*. Celiac disease can be found in all ages, races, and ethnicities. About 10% to 20% of close relatives of people with celiac disease also are affected.[8]

It seems that celiac disease can develop in a person at risk at any time. There are 3 factors that come together to cause celiac disease.

1. Overresponsive immune system
2. Genetic predisposition
3. Factors in an individual environment[6]

DISCUSSION

Some individuals can eat gluten for 50 years and then develop celiac disease, whereas others can be diagnosed in 9 months of eating gluten. Many have silent celiac disease, which means that symptoms are absent in them but they are not necessarily healthy. Therefore it is imperative to be diagnosed early. Early diagnosis can prevent the development of other autoimmune disorders and additional complications. Regular antibody testing is key to diagnosis.[11]

Clinical manifestations and symptoms of celiac disease include gastrointestinal symptoms, extraintestinal presentations, autoimmune disorders, biliary disorders, and inflammatory and miscellaneous conditions.[12] Gastrointestinal symptoms include heartburn, dyspepsia, nausea, vomiting, steatorrhea, abdominal pain, and irritable bowel syndrome. Extraintestinal symptoms include iron and folate deficiency, osteopenia, dermatitis herpetiform, fatigue, infertility, and aphthous stomatitis.[12] Autoimmune disorders include diabetes, thyroid and adrenal disease, Sjögren syndrome, rheumatoid arthritis, and systemic lupus erythematosus.[12]

Biliary disorders include cholangitis, cirrhosis, and elevated aminotransferase levels.[12]

Inflammatory disorders include microscopic colitis, inflammatory bowel disease, and gastritis.[12] Miscellaneous disorders include IgA deficiency, IgA nephropathy, Down syndrome, and Turner syndrome.[12]

Physical findings include muscle wasting, pallor, bruising, edema stomatitis, aphthous ulcerations, cheilosis, vertebral fractures, tetany finger clubbing, protuberant abdomen, short stature, and dental enamel defects.[12] Common conditions or disorders associated with celiac disease include diabetes, Down syndrome, dermatitis herpetiformis, hypothyroidism/hyperthyroidism, rheumatoid arthritis, microscopic colitis, irritable bowel syndrome, pancreatic insufficiency, IgA deficiency, autoimmune liver disease, and intestinal lymphoma.[12]

Who Should Be Tested?

1. Children older than 3 years and adults experiencing symptoms of celiac disease should be tested.[13]
2. First-degree relatives of people with celiac disease, parents, siblings, and children have a 1 in 10 risk compared with 1 in 100 risk in the general population.[13]
3. Any individual with an associated autoimmune disorder or other condition especially type 1 diabetes mellitus, autoimmune thyroid disease, autoimmune liver disease, Down syndrome, Turner syndrome, Williams syndrome, and selective immunoglobulin IgA deficiency.[13]
4. Children older than 3 years and adults regardless of symptoms if related to a close relative (parent, sibling, or child) with biopsy-confirmed celiac disease.[4]

5. Children younger than 3 years should be evaluated by a pediatric gastroenterologist. Generally speaking, children should be eating wheat rye or barley up to 1 year before being tested to generate an autoimmune response to gluten.[4]
6. Any individual who has a related autoimmune disorder, regardless of celiac symptoms, and retested periodically. These conditions consist of insulin-dependent diabetes mellitus, Hashimoto thyroiditis, Down syndrome, Turner syndrome, Williams syndrome, Grave disease, and Sjögren disease.[4]
7. Anyone who has experienced persistent miscarriage or infertility where a medical cause could not be found needs to be tested.[4]
8. Those with other conditions such as persistent gastrointestinal symptoms, bone density problems, dental enamel hypoplasia, and fatigue should be tested.[4]

The differential diagnosis for celiac disease includes inflammatory bowel disease, microscopic colitis, lactose intolerance, irritable bowel syndrome, pancreatic insufficiency, nonceliac gluten sensitivity, small intestinal bacterial overgrowth, Giardia infection, IgA deficiency, common variable immunodeficiency (CVID), and eosinophilic gastroenteritis.[12]

Celiac disease is challenging to diagnose because there are so many conditions to consider. Physicians do not routinely test for celiac disease. However, if family members have celiac disease with type 1 diabetes, this may point providers to screen for this disease. Researchers recommend routine screening of all family members (parents and sibling) for celiac disease.[9] The diagnosis is made by family history, physical examination, and tests. Tests include blood tests, genetic markers, and small bowel biopsy.[9]

Some common physical examination findings include rash, malnutrition, abdominal sounds, pain with palpation, abdominal fullness, and dental examination for yellow or brown spots on teeth.

Diagnostic testing includes complete blood cell count (CBC), iron, ferritin, liver function test, vitamin D, vitamin B_1, vitamin B_6, thiamine, calcium, zinc, copper, thyroid function tests, and bone density.[12]

In patients with celiac disease, nutritional markers should be evaluated at diagnosis, and abnormal findings should be reassessed after 1 year of adherence to a gluten-free diet. Up to 28% of children presenting with celiac disease have a nutritional deficiency, such as iron (28%), folate (14%), vitamin B_{12} (1%), or vitamin D (27%) deficiency at diagnosis.[14,15]

Children's growth should be routinely monitored. Current guidelines recommend follow-up serologic testing to assess dietary adherence and for use as a surrogate marker of mucosal recovery in children and adults.[14] Adults presenting with celiac disease are likely to have a nutritional deficiency, such as folate (20%), B_{12} (19%), or zinc (67%), and iron deficiency anemia (32%).[16]

Serologic tests for celiac disease provide an effective first step in identifying individuals for intestinal biopsy. If a serologic or genetic test indicates the possibility of celiac disease, a biopsy should be done promptly and before initiating any dietary changes. Genetic tests that confirm the presence or absence of specific genes associated with celiac disease may be beneficial in some cases. A biopsy is important because without a definitive diagnostic test patients who are conformed to have celiac disease are less likely to adhere to a strict gluten-free diet.[9]

Researchers have discovered that people with celiac disease and eat gluten have higher levels of specific antibodies in their bloods. These antibodies are products of the immune system in response to substances that the body perceives as a threat. Antibodies that are produced when consuming gluten include anti-tTG antibodies, endomysial antibodies (EMA), and DGP antibodies.[9]

Anti-Tissue Transglutaminase Antibodies

Anti-tTG antibodies are commonly tested when an individual is in a high-risk group for celiac disease (whether or not the person has symptoms). Testing for these antibodies is the most sensitive test available.[11]

The tTg-IgA test is an enzyme-linked immunosorbent assay (ELISA). The tTG-IgA test is the preferred screening method and has a sensitivity of 95%, yielding few false-negative results. The tTG test also has a specificity of more than 96%. This test can be used to assess initiation and maintenance of a gluten-free diet. The test may be less sensitive among people with milder celiac disease depending on the degree of intestinal damage.[9]

Endomysial Antibodies

EMA test has a specificity of 98%, making it the most specific test for celiac disease, although it is not as sensitive as the tTG-IgA test.[17] The test has a sensitivity of 90%, which may be due in part to the high technical difficulty in performing the test. EMA are measured by indirect immunofluorescent assay; it is a more expensive and time-consuming process then ELISA. In addition, the EMA test is qualitative, making the result more subjective than that for tTG- IgA. EMA test is often used as an adjunctive test to the routine tTG-IgA test.[18]

If tTG-TgA or EMA-IgA test result is negative and celiac disease is still suspected, total IgA should be measured to identify selective IgA deficiency. This condition can cause a false-negative test result.

Total Serum IgA

Total serum IgA level is used to check for IgA deficiency. IgA deficiency is diagnosed when someone has a total serum IgA test and the result is close to 0; this is not a test for celiac disease but a means of making a more accurate diagnosis.[11] IgA deficiency affects 2% to 3% of patients with celiac disease or people who test negative for tTG-IgA or EMA. IgA deficiency in a patient may indicate other diseases that may cause villus atrophy, such as giardiasis, small bowel bacterial overgrowth, or CVID.[17] It is possible to have a negative antibody test result and still have celiac disease. IgA deficiency is one example of when this might occur.[11] tTG antibodies and EMA are IgA based. If an IgA-deficient patient is tested for these IgA-based antibodies the test result will be negative because the patient has no IgA to be detected. This will result in a false-negative result. The tTG-TgG test is *only* useful in those subjects who have an IgA deficiency, which is 1 in 400 of the general population or 2% or 3% of people with celiac disease.[19] The most sensitive antibody test is the immunoglobulin A (IgA) test. However, immunoglobulin G (IgG) tests may be used in people with IgA deficiency.[9]

Deamidated Gliadin Peptide Antibodies

In cases of tTG-IgA deficiency, tTG-IgG or DGP-IgG should be used to measure antibody level. DGP-IgG has reasonable sensitivity for celiac disease in IgA-sufficient and IgA-deficient patients.[9]

A positive result of tTG-IGA, EMA, or DGP-IgG antibody test indicates that the person needs to have a biopsy to confirm the diagnosis of celiac disease. A positive antibody test result does not reflect a positive celiac disease diagnosis. The endoscopic biopsy obtains a small piece of tissue from the small intestines in 5 to 6 areas of the small intestines. This biopsy examines areas of the bowel for damage to the villi and is the gold standard for diagnosing celiac disease.[11]

For accurate diagnostic test results, patients must be on a gluten-containing diet.[9]

Sensitivity Versus Specificity

Sensitivity: refers to how correctly the test identifies those with the disease. The tTG-IgA test will give positive result in about 98% of patients with celiac disease who are on a gluten-containing diet. The same test will give negative result in about 95% of healthy people without celiac disease.[17]

Specificity: refers to how accurately the test is able to identify those without the disease. The tTG test is the most sensitive test for celiac disease.[5]

Genetic Testing

Human leukocyte antigens (HLA-DQ2 and HLA-DQ8) are genetic markers used to determine if a patient could develop celiac disease. These are not antibody tests. Carrying HLA DQ2 and/or HLA DQ8 is neither a diagnosis of celiac disease nor does it mean that one will ever develop celiac disease.[20] These antigens are used to exclude celiac disease; if the test result is negative then it is doubtful the patient has or will develop celiac disease. Most people with celiac disease have gene pairs that encode for at least one of the HLA gene variants, or alleles, designated HLA-DQ2, found in 95% of people with disease, and HLA-DQ8. However, these alleles are found in about 30% to 35% Caucasians and most people with the variants do not develop celiac disease.[21]

HLA testing checks for genetic mutations related to celiac disease. These mutations include HLA-DQ2 and HLA-DQ8. Specific variations in HLA alleles (HLA-DQ) predispose one to celiac disease. More than 90% of people with celiac disease have the HLA-DQ2 while a small percentage has the HLA-DQ8. The primary use of these celiac HLA-DQ markers is to determine if one has or is genetically susceptible to celiac disease. This type of genetic typing is helpful if one has had a small bowel biopsy with indeterminate results or before committing to a gluten-free diet. In other circumstances, celiac genetic testing may avoid the need for a biopsy in people who have a high likelihood of being positive. Celiac laboratory results that are negative for both HLA-DQ2 and HLA-DQ8, in most cases, will exclude the diagnosis of celiac disease and the possibility of getting it in the future. A positive DQ2 or DQ8 laboratory test result, particularly when found with suspicious biopsy results, is typically considered positive for celiac disease. Although up to 40% of the population carries the genotype HLA-DQ2 or HLA-DQ8, required for the development of celiac disease, only 2% to 3% of HLA-DQ2 or HLA-DQ8 carriers subsequently develop celiac disease.[22] Research suggests that celiac disease only develops in individuals who have these particular genes.[23]

As celiac disease is genetic, this means it runs in the families. First-degree family members (parents, siblings, and children) who have the same genotype as the family member with celiac disease, have up to a 40% risk of developing celiac disease. The overall risk of developing celiac disease when the genotype is 7% to 20%.[20]

Negative findings for HLA-DQ2 and HLA-DQ8 make current or future celiac disease unlikely in patients for whom other tests, including biopsy, do not provide a clear diagnostic result.[24]

Clinically, genetic testing for *HLA-DQ2* and *HLA-DQ8* may be helpful to determine whether patients in high-risk groups, such as family members or patients with comorbid conditions such as autoimmune thyroid disease, need screening for celiac disease. Genetic testing also may be used for patients already following a gluten-free diet who have not been accurately assessed for celiac disease and are hesitant to reintroduce gluten into their diet for an accurate diagnostic reevaluation. In these cases, if patients do not carry the *HLA-DQ2* or *HLA-DQ8* genes, they would not require further diagnostic workup to evaluate for celiac disease.[24]

Who Should Have Human Leucocyte Antigen Antigen Testing?

Patients who should have HLA antigen testing include those who have been on a gluten-free diet and antibody blood testing is not accurate, those who have an unclear diagnosis of celiac disease, or those who have a family member who has been diagnosed with celiac disease.[22]

In addition, a negative HLA antigen test result assures a 99% probability that the family member will *not* develop celiac disease and a positive result indicates the family member should follow-up with celiac antibody testing every 2 to 3 years or immediately if symptoms develop.[22]

What Is the Gold Standard for Diagnosing Celiac Disease?

Small intestinal biopsy (endoscopic duodenal mucosal biopsy) is historically known as the gold standard for diagnosing celiac disease. However, highly sensitive and specific serologic tests have been used for screening patients for celiac disease. At present, there is no serologic test available with 100% sensitivity and specificity, and therefore a biopsy is necessary for a definitive diagnosis. It is important that this test is performed while the patient is on a regular, gluten-containing diet.

An endoscopic examination of the mucosa of the small bowel of a patient with celiac disease may demonstrate villi absent or atrophic. Often there is crypt hyperplasia present with lymphocytes and plasma cells seen in the lamina propria.[25]

Management Plan for Celiac Disease

At the time of diagnosis the provider should:

1. Perform a complete physical examination including body mass index and examination of lymph nodes and occult blood in the stool.
2. Perform bone densitometry for severe malabsorption or bone health issues
3. Perform celiac serology (anti-DGP IgA and anti-tTG IgA) and DQ2 and DQ8 genetic testing
4. Perform blood tests: CBC, iron studies, vitamin B studies, thyroid function tests with thyrotropin, liver enzymes, and calcium, phosphate, 25-hydroxyvitamin D, copper, and zinc levels.
5. Recommend family screening (DQ2 and DQ8 genetic testing and celiac serology including anti-tTG IgA, anti-DP IgG, and total IgA deficiency)
6. Consult dietician to provide education and counseling
7. Consult mental health professional to address psychosocial aspect of going gluten free and coping with a chronic disease
8. Recommend a gluten-free multivitamin
9. Assess hepatitis B, flu, and pneumococcal immunization status

It is important to identify and treat nutritional deficiencies. Patients diagnosed with celiac disease will be referred to a dietitian who specializes in treating people with celiac disease.[9] It is recommended that everyone who is diagnosed with celiac disease follow a strict gluten-free diet. Most people who follow a gluten-free diet improve within days to weeks, and most will heal damage in the small intestines and prevent more damage.[9] The small intestine usually heals in 3 to 6 months in children. Complete healing can take several years in adults. Once the intestine heals the villi, which were damaged by the disease, regrow and will absorb nutrients from food into the bloodstream normally.[9]

The gluten-free diet allows for healing of the villous atrophy in the small intestine, causing symptoms to resolve. Following a gluten-free diet also helps prevent future complications including malignancies.

In patients with celiac disease, nutritional markers should be evaluated at diagnosis and abnormal findings should be reassessed after 1 year of adherence to a gluten-free diet. Up to 28% of children presenting with celiac disease have a nutritional deficiency, such as iron (28%), folate (14%), vitamin B_{12} (1%), or vitamin D (27%) deficiency, at diagnosis.[9] Adults presenting with celiac disease are likely to have a nutritional deficiency, such as folate (20%), B_{12} (19%), or zinc (67%) and iron deficiency (32%).[26] Children's growth should be routinely monitored. Current guidelines recommend follow-up serologic testing to assess dietary adherence and for use as a surrogate marker of mucosal recovery in children and adults.[26]

Vitamin dietary supplements may be necessary because many people with celiac disease are deficient in fiber, iron, calcium, magnesium, zinc, folate, niacin, riboflavin, vitamin B_{12}, and vitamin D as well as in calories and protein. Deficiencies in copper and vitamin B_6 are also possible but less common. Deficiencies in B_{12} and folate may help patients with celiac disease who have anxiety and depression caused by vitamin deficiencies.[13]

Patients with celiac disease should be followed up closely for dietary adherence, nutritional deficiencies, and the development of possible comorbidities. Follow-up testing is conducted to ensure that antibody levels are returning to normal, indicating that the intestine is healing on the new diet. For this reason repeated intestinal biopsies are no longer necessary. These tests also indicate the extent to which a celiac is avoiding gluten and can detect when hidden gluten has entered the diet.[11]

Follow-up should occur twice in the first year of diagnosis. The first appointment should be 3 to 6 months after the initial visit, and the second visit should be after 1 year on the gluten-free diet. After that the celiac should receive follow-up testing on a yearly basis.[11]

Follow-up is important because it can raise awareness to any health concerns that may come up (joint pain, rash). Follow-up will ensure that the gluten-free diet is working or if changes need to be made to ensure health. Negative results reinforce the family's approach to a gluten-free diet and that it is working well. Negative results indicate strong level of compliance with the diet and it is unlikely that celiac disease is contributing to new condition. Although it is not an exact science, follow-up testing can often clarify that a new health condition could be a complication of celiac disease.[11] A repeat bone densitometry is recommended at 2 to 3 years, if previously abnormal and for adolescents noncompliant with gluten-free diet. In addition, a repeat small intestinal biopsy is recommended at 3 to 5 years to assess dietary compliance and to rule out refractory celiac disease. Celiac-specific autoantibody levels should be measured every 6 to 12 months after initiation of the gluten-free diet until they normalize.[3,26]

Unresponsive patients need to be monitored and assessed for compliance with the diet. Serology testing can assess compliance. Noncompliance can be unintentional in an individual who may be still ingesting gluten without realizing.[27,28]

It is estimated that up to 30% of patients with celiac disease have persistent symptoms while on a gluten-free diet.[13] The most common reason for persistent symptoms is continuing to ingest gluten either knowingly or unknowingly. Patients are encouraged to meet with a dietitian to learn about "hidden" sources of gluten.[29] Recommendations also support a baseline dual-energy x-ray absorptiometry scan for women and men older than 30 years diagnosed with celiac disease.[30] All patients should be prescribed 1200 mg calcium and 800 IU vitamin D daily. Each patient should receive the pneumococcal and flu vaccine.

A negative genetic marker gene test result excludes the possibility of later developing celiac disease, so this can be valuable information for first-degree family members. It is recommended that genetic testing for celiac disease be completed on all family members, especially children, to prevent future unnecessary testing. Screening gene-positive first-degree relatives every 3 to 5 years is recommended.[13]

Dietary management: Patients should avoid all products that contain gluten, such as most cereal, grains, and pasta and many processed foods.[31] Reading all food labels is critical for success. Patients should discuss gluten-free options with a dietician or health care professional who specializes in celiac disease. Meat, corn, quinoa, buck wheat, millet, fish, fruits, vegetables, rice, and potatoes without additives or seasonings are safe for patients to eat. Gluten-free bread, pasta, and other gluten-free foods are also safe options. Potatoes, rice, soy, amaranth, quinoa, buckwheat, or bean flour instead of wheat flour are approved for patients with celiac on a gluten-free diet. Oats are safe as long as they do not come in contact with wheat gluten during processing.[9]

Gluten sometimes appears in foods or places in which one would not ordinarily suspect; these can include but are not limited to:

1. Thickening agent in many gravies and sauces
2. Medications, vitamins, and supplements
3. Lip balm, lipstick, and other cosmetics

It is important when preparing gluten-free foods to prevent cross-contamination with foods containing gluten. Cross-contamination can occur if foods are prepared on common surfaces or with utensils that are not thoroughly cleaned after preparing gluten-containing foods.[32] Using hard-to-clean equipment for both gluten-free and gluten-containing foods is often a source of contamination. Toasters, strainers, and flour sifters should not be shared. Deep-fried foods cooked in oil also used to cook breaded products should not be used.

Spreadable condiments in shared containers may also be a source of contamination. When a person dips into a condiment such as mustard, mayonnaise, jam, peanut butter, or margarine a second time with the knife used for spreading, the condiment becomes contaminated with crumbs and is not safe for consumption by individuals who cannot tolerate gluten. Consider using condiments in squeeze containers to prevent cross-contamination. Wheat flour can stay airborne for many hours in a bakery or in a home and contaminate exposed preparation surfaces and utensils or uncovered gluten-free products.[32]

SUMMARY

Celiac disease is a chronic autoimmune disease, which means one cannot "grow out" of it. The treatment of celiac disease is a lifelong adherence to a strict gluten-free diet. Only food and beverage with gluten content less than 20 ppm is allowed.[13]

Effective screening methods, early identification, diagnosis, and management are critical in effectively treating and avoiding long-term complications in patients with celiac disease. Celiac disease was once known as the zebra. Health care providers have come a long way in exploring the causes, pathogenesis, and treatment of celiac disease. The treatment of celiac disease is a lifelong commitment to a strict gluten-free diet. Adjusting to this lifelong commitment can have negative effects on a patient's quality of life.

Adhering to a gluten-free diet is often difficult in the first year of being diagnosed. Some patients experience social isolation, anxiety, and depression. Gluten-free food can be quite costly, especially if patients are eating out. Patients run the risk of cross-contamination with food preparation. Some restaurants are not fully educated on what is celiac disease and what are the risks of intestinal damage.

What Are the Challenges of a Diagnosis of Celiac Disease

1. Celiac disease affects all walks of life. What used to be seen as a childhood disease is now seen in all ages across the life span.
2. Celiac disease awareness in food restaurants
3. Limited food options within the community and resources.
4. Celiac disease awareness among hospital personnel and dietary services
5. Patient education on compliancy and lifelong treatment.
6. Early and proper identification of celiac disease.
7. The average number of years to obtain a diagnosis is 11 years.[32]

The gluten-free diet is a lifelong commitment and should not be started before being properly diagnosed. Starting a diet without a complete workup and testing is not recommended and makes later diagnosis difficult.[32] Tests to confirm celiac disease could be falsely negative if a person were on a gluten-free diet for a period before testing. For a valid diagnosis to be made, gluten would need to be reintroduced for at least several weeks before testing.[32]

Implementation of the gluten-free diet is the only treatment of celiac disease and therefore acts to prevent possible morbidity and mortality associated with untreated celiac disease.[24]

The implementation of a gluten-free diet in patients with celiac disease may be associated with a protective effect against autoimmune disease such as thyroid disease.[33] The goals for treating a patient with celiac disease include improving symptoms, improving quality of life, avoiding complications, normalizing celiac antibodies, and facilitating small bowel healing.

Important Things to Remember

1. A gluten-free diet is a lifelong commitment and the basis of treatment of celiac disease.
2. Registered dietician nutritionist should be involved in the education of the patient and family members.
3. Nutritional supplements may be needed: iron, vitamin D, and other vitamins and minerals.
4. Lack of response to gluten-free diet should be a red flag to the health care provider. The provider must consider unintended gluten ingestion.
5. Other comorbid conditions must be considered if gluten-free diet is ineffective and/or possible incorrect diagnosis.
6. Refractory celiac disease and/or lymphoma must be considered.
7. Gastroenterologist may need to be consulted.

CLINICS CARE POINTS

- Endoscopic biopsy is the gold standard for diagnosing celiac disease.
- Patients are advised not to start a gluten-free diet before the diagnosis has been confirmed.
- Clinicians must identify IgA-deficient patients to properly diagnosis celiac disease.
- Positive result for genetic markers does not mean positive for celiac disease

- A biopsy is important because without a definitive diagnostic test confirming celiac disease patients are less likely to adhere to a strict gluten-free diet.

DISCLOSURE

The author has nothing to disclose.

REFERENCES

1. Ludvigsson JF, Lefler DA, Bai JC, et al. The Oslo definitions for coeliac disease and related terms. Gut 2013;62(1):43–52.
2. Holmes G. History of coeliac disease. Coeliac UK. Archived from the original on 12 March 2007. 2006. Available at: http://www.coeliac.co.uk/coeliac_disease/68.asp. Accessed March 23, 2007.
3. Rubio-Tapia A, Hill ID, Kelly CP, et al. ACG Clinical Guidelines: diagnosis and management of celiac disease. Am J Gastroenterol 2013;108(5):656–76.
4. Celiac Disease Screening. Medlinelineplus.gove website. Available at: https://medlineplus.gov/celiacdisease.html#cat. Access November 12, 2020.
5. Celiac Disease. Family doctor website. Available at: https://familydoctor.org/condition/celiac-disease/?adfree=true. Accessed November 12, 2020.
6. Gujral N, Freeman HJ, Thomson AB. Celiac disease: prevalence, diagnosis, pathogenesis and treatment. World J Gastroenterol 2012;18:6036–59.
7. Celiac Disease. Clinical features, diagnosis and management. Available at: http://www.utube.com/watch?v=U9qhihsEOcQ. Accessed December 5, 2020.
8. Celiac Disease. Medlineplus.gov website. Available at: https://medlineplus.gov/celiacdisease.html#cat. Accessed November 12, 2020.
9. Celiac Disease – Definition and Facts. NIDDK.NIH website. Available at: https://www.niddk.nih.gov/health-information/digestive-diseases/celiac-disease. Accessed November 6, 2020.
10. Faso A, Berti I, Gerarduzzi T, et al. Prevalence of celiac disease in at-risk and not-at-risk groups in the United States: a large multicenter study. Arch Intern Med 2003;163(3):286–92.
11. Symptoms. University of Chicago – Celiac Disease Center Website. Available at: http://www.cureceliacdisease.org/wp-content/uploads/341_CDCFACTSHEET2_Symptoms.pdf. Accessed November 6, 2020.
12. Rubin J, Crowe S. In the Clinic – Celiac Disease, Annals of Internal Medicine in the Clinic, January 7, 2020, 1-16. 2020. Available at: https://www.acpjournals.org/doi/10.7326/AITC202001070.
13. Testing. Celiac Disease Foundation. Available at: https://celiac.org/about-celiac-disease/screening-and-diagnosis/screening/. Accessed November 6, 2020.
14. Wessels MM, van Veen II, Vriezinga SL, et al. Complementary serologic investigations in children with celiac disease is unnecessary during follow-up. J Pediatr 2016;169:55–60.
15. Husby S, Koletzko S, Korponay-Szabó IR, et al, ESPGHAN Working Group on Coeliac Disease Diagnosis, ESPGHAN Gastroenterology Committee, European Society for Pediatric Gastroenterology, Hepatology, and Nutrition. European Society for Pediatric Gastroenterology, Hepatology, and Nutrition guidelines for the diagnosis of coeliac disease. J Pediatr Gastroenterol Nutr 2012;54(1):136–60.

16. Wierdsma NJ, van Bokhorst-de van der Schueren MA, Berkenpas M, et al. Vitamin and mineral deficiencies are highly prevalent in newly diagnosed celiac disease patients. Nutrients 2013;5(10):3975–92.
17. Al-Toma A, Volta U, Auricchio R, et al. European Society for the Study of Coeliac Disease (ESsCD) guideline for coeliac disease and other gluten-related disorders. United European Gastroenterol J 2019;7(5):583–613.
18. Wenzl TG, Benninga MA, Loots CM, et al, ESPGHAN EURO-PIG Working Group. Indications, methodology, and interpretation of combined esophageal impedance-pH monitoring in children: ESPGHAN EURO-PIG standard protocol. J Pediatr Gastroenterol Nutr 2012;55(2):230–4.
19. Chow MA, Lebwohl B, Reilly NR, et al. Immunoglobulin A deficiency in celiac disease. J Clin Gastroenterol 2012;46(10):850–4.
20. Testing. Celiac Disease Foundation website. Available at: https://celiac.org/about-celiac-disease/screening-and-diagnosis/screening/. Accessed November 6, 2020.
21. Scanlon SA, Murray JA. Update on celiac disease—etiology, differential diagnosis, drug targets, and management advances. Clin Exp Gastroenterol 2011;4.
22. Leonard MM, Serena G, Sturgeon C, et al. Genetics and celiac disease: the importance of screening. Exp Rev Gastroenterol Hepatol 2015;9(2):209–15.
23. Celiac Disease. Medlineplus website. Available at: https://medlineplus.gov/celiacdisease.html#cat_95. Accessed November 6, 2020.
24. Available at: https://jamanetwork-com.ezproxy-v.musc.edu/journals/jama/fullarticle/2648637.
25. Bai JC, Ciacci C. World Gastroenterology Organisation Global Guidelines: Celiac Disease February 2017. J Clin Gastroenterol 2017;51(9):755–68.
26. Hill ID, Dirks MH, Liptak GS, et al, North American Society for Pediatric Gastroenterology, Hepatology and Nutrition. Guideline for the diagnosis and treatment of celiac disease in children: recommendations of the North American Society for Pediatric Gastroenterology, Hepatology and Nutrition. J Pediatr Gastroenterol Nutr 2005;40(1):1–19.
27. Walker MM, Ludvigsson JF, Sanders DS. Coeliac disease: review of diagnosis and management. Med J Aust 2017;207(4):173–8.
28. Werkstetter KJ, Korponay-Szabo IR, Popp A, et al, ProCeDE study group. Accuracy in diagnosis of celiac disease without biopsies in clinical practice. Gastroenterology 2017;153(4):924–35.
29. Pietzak MM. Follow-up of patients with celiac disease: achieving compliance with treatment. Gastroenterology 2005;128(4 suppl 1):S135–41.
30. Pantaleoni S, Luchino M, Adriani A, et al. Bone mineral density at diagnosis of celiac disease and after 1 year of gluten-free diet. ScientificWorldJournal 2014;2014:173082.
31. Celiac Disease. Gikids website. Available at: https://gikids.org/celiac-disease/. Accessed November 2, 2020.
32. Getting Started on a Gluten Free Diet. Gluten Intolerance Website. 2019. https://gluten.org/2019/12/14/getting-started-on-a-gluten-free-diet/. Accessed November 2, 2020.
33. Cosnes J, Cellier C, Viola S, et al. Groupe D'Etude et de Recherche Sur la Maladie Coeliaque. Incidence of autoimmune diseases in celiac disease: protective effect of the gluten-free diet. Clin Gastroenterol Hepatol 2008;6(7):753–8.

Evaluating Patients for Nutritional Deficiencies

Tenell Zahodnik, MPAS, PA-C, CAQ-EM

KEYWORDS

- Nutritional deficiencies • Vitamins • Minerals • Fat soluble • Water soluble
- Special populations

KEY POINTS

- Nutritional deficiencies are common in adults and children globally.
- Clinicians can use history and physical examination to identify potential deficiencies in their patients.
- New prevention solutions can help to avoid long-term sequelae.

INTRODUCTION

Nutritional deficiencies have significant morbidity and mortality with the World Health Organization (WHO) reporting that close to 2 billion people around the globe are at risk for such deficiencies.[1] Malnutrition has been defined as the body not receiving enough nutrients to maintain a healthy state or as a loss of body weight or mass, whether that lack of mass is categorized by a loss of fat or muscle.[2] The lack of proper nutrition can be broken down into minerals versus vitamins, with the vitamins category further broken down into 2 smaller subsets of water soluble or fat soluble[3,4] (**Table 1**). Whether a vitamin is fat or water soluble is determined by how it is absorbed and stored in the body.[4] We as humans cannot synthesize vitamins and therefore rely on our diet or supplements to ensure that we are getting adequate amounts to maintain a state of health[3] (**Table 2**). Each of these individual deficiencies has a multitude of data and details; this article gives an overview of a variety of these issues to provide general understanding.

WATER SOLUBLE

As their title implies, water-soluble vitamins are quickly dissolved into water once they enter the body and are therefore not easily stored in the body.[4] The B vitamins, of which there are 8 specific ones, and vitamin C fall into this category. A discussion of the B vitamins is outside the scope of this work. The most commonly found deficiencies are discussed.

Department of Physician Assistant Studies, Hardin-Simmons University, 2200 Hickory Street, HSU Box 16236, Abilene, TX 79698, USA
E-mail address: tenell.zahodnik@hsutx.edu

Physician Assist Clin 6 (2021) 581–592
https://doi.org/10.1016/j.cpha.2021.05.003
2405-7991/21/© 2021 Elsevier Inc. All rights reserved.

Table 1 Water-soluble versus fat-soluble vitamins	
Water-Soluble Vitamins	**Fat-Soluble Vitamins**
Vitamin B1 (thiamine)	Vitamin A
Vitamin B2[a]	Vitamin D
Vitamin B3 (niacin)	Vitamin E[a]
Vitamin B6[a]	Vitamin K[a]
Vitamin B12	
Vitamin B9 (folate)	
Vitamin B7 (biotin)[a]	
Pantothenate[a]	
Vitamin C	

[a] Vitamins not covered in this article.

Vitamin B1

Vitamin B1, otherwise known as thiamine, is particularly important for cognitive and cardiac health, and inadequate amounts of this vitamin can result in significant consequences for individuals. The human body is only capable of storing approximately 25 to 30 mg thiamine at a time, and currently it is recommended that 1 to 1.5 mg thiamine should be ingested daily by way of diet.[5] Thiamine deficiency has been given the name "beriberi" with 2 clinical categories including dry and wet beriberi.[6] The most simplistic way to think about these deficiencies is to think of dry beriberi relating to the nervous system with manifestations of such and for wet beriberi to have cardiac manifestations.[5-7] Wet beriberi's cardiac issues can range from peripheral edema to heart failure, whereas dry beriberi manifestations range from pain, peripheral neuropathies, and loss of reflexes.[6] In dry beriberi, the lower extremities tend to be affected more than the upper extremities with regard to these sensory changes.[5,6] When severe deficiencies are encountered, dry beriberi can progress to Wernicke encephalopathy (WE) and Korsakoff syndrome (KS).[6,8] Historically, patients with WE were thought to present with a triad of findings that included changes in mental status, nystagmus due to weakening of the eye muscles, and ataxia in their gait. Searching for this triad clinically can be misleading because only one-tenth of cases are thought to present with the full triad of symptoms.[7-9] A helpful pneumonic to aid a practitioner in identifying which patient might be at risk is *WACO* to stand for Wernicke ataxia, confusion, and ophthalmoplegia.[9] Patients with the most severe cases of thiamine deficiency then progress on to the next stage, that is, KS. It is estimated that approximately 80% of patients with WE progress to KS and will show additional findings of amnesia and confabulation.[6,8]

Initial treatment has historically been 100 mg intramuscular thiamine; however, there is debate as to if this dosage is enough for patients with WE and KS presentations, indicating severe deficiencies.[8] Some studies show that as much as 500 mg intravenous thiamine is required 3 times a day for 3 days before patients can be switched to an oral formulation that is weight based.[6,9] Long-term supplementation is typically required.

Vitamin B3

Vitamin B3 is otherwise known as niacin. Inadequate amounts of B3 can cause a condition called pellagra. This condition is associated with a collection of findings often

Table 2	
Naturally occurring sources of vitamins	
Water Soluble	**Sources**
B1, thiamine	Squash, green peas, quinoa, pork, oatmeal, trout, sunflower seeds, cereals, brown rice
B2, riboflavin	Eggs, milk, mushrooms, spinach, raspberries, liver
B3, niacin	Kidney beans, broccoli, chicken fish tomatoes
B5, pantothenate	Pork, avocado, sweet potatoes, corn, chicken liver, broccoli, egg yolk, cauliflower
B6, pyridoxine, pyridoxal	Bananas, avocado, cabbage, soy milk, chicken breast, sunflower seeds
B7, biotin	Romaine lettuce, salmon, egg yolks, beef liver, carrots, grapefruit, oats, walnuts
B9, folate	Spinach, brussels sprouts, beef liver, okra, bell pepper, beets, mustard greens, oranges
B12, cobalamin	Sardines, clams, eggs, liver, low-fat milk, fortified cereals, king crab
Vitamin C	Oranges, limes, melon, strawberries, broccoli, peppers, brussels sprouts, kale, tomatoes, spinach
Fat Soluble	**Sources**
Vitamin A	Carrots, pumpkin, red bell pepper, mango, broccoli, sweet potato, avocado
Vitamin D	Mushrooms, fish, eggs, fortified cereals, broccoli, carrots, peppers
Vitamin E	Almonds, Swiss chard, avocado, olive oil, sunflower seeds, trout, corn, green olives
Vitamin K	Kale, brussels sprouts, asparagus, spinach, green pears, parsley, kiwi broccoli

alluded to as the "4 Ds," which stand for diarrhea, dermatitis, dementia, and death if no intervention is undertaken.[10] In regard to the *D* of dermatitis, individuals with B3 deficiency will have hyperpigmented areas of the skin that are most readily exposed to the sun, for example, the dorsum of the hands, feet, and the neck.[11] The diarrhea these patients experience can be severe enough to cause the intestinal villi to atrophy and increase their chances of malabsorption, only magnifying their current problem.[6] Treatment of these patients entails oral replenishment of niacin, typically 100 mg every 6 hours until the bulk of symptoms subside; for patients with cutaneous findings a longer course is necessary with 50 mg of niacin by mouth every 8 to 12 hours until the skin heals.[9]

Vitamin B9

Vitamin B9, folate, plays an important role of development in fetuses, most notably with the neural tube formation.[12] Within the first 4 to 6 weeks of conception, the neural tube forms in the embryo and will eventually close to form the fetus' brain and spinal cord.[13] A malformation of the neural tube causes devastating defects that can include anencephaly or spina bifida.[14] Given that often early pregnancy may not be recognized until after this critical window of development, it is now recommended that women of child-bearing status make a minimum 400 μg folate a part of their daily intake to prevent such detrimental birth defects.[13] The need for all women who are capable of reproducing to modify their diets is supported by the fact that approximately half of the pregnancies in the United States alone are not planned for.[14] The US Food and Drug Administration attempted to alleviate some of this burden in 1998 by having flours "enriched" with folate to help women achieve proper levels to avoid neural tube defects.[12,13]

Vitamin B12

Vitamin B12 is in the family of cobalamins, and all cells in the body use it.[15] Daily utilization of B12 usually falls within the 3 to 5 μg range, and the liver is the primary place of storage with approximate 2 to 5 mg deposited at a given time.[6] The most common manifestation of B12 deficiency is megaloblastic anemia with other signs and symptoms landing on a spectrum from mild fatigue to neuropathy, or even bouts of psychosis.[16] Studies have also shown that B12 plays a crucial role in infants' central nervous system development because it is thought that B12 aids in myelination and early brain development.[12] During gestation, vitamin B12 is stored in the fetus' liver, and this should be an adequate amount of storage for the infant's first 4 months of life.[12] Deficiency is most likely identified somewhere in the first 2 to 12 months, and this is often associated with breastfeeding from a mom who is deficient herself at baseline or who adheres to a vegan or vegetarian diet.[17,18] Infants who are deficient in vitamin B12 are found to have a range of findings with the most severe showing brain atrophy.[12]

Our understanding of how vitamins and nutrition play into our well-being is expanding every day. An example of this is in the coronavirus disease 2019 (COVID-19) virus. The world continues to reel from its emergence and the devastation it caused. It has been documented that this novel virus disproportionately affects the elderly population and diabetics.[19] The elderly are already at risk for B12 deficiency with some estimates that 20% of the population that is 60 years or older residing in the United States or United Kingdom is deficient.[16] In addition, diabetic patients on metfomin are often deficient in B12 at baseline.[20] There is new research looking into how elderly and diabetic patients who contract COVID-19 might be treated, delving into the possibility of vitamin B12 serving as an adjunct therapy.[16,19] Some of the data that have recently been reported on this topic show that B12 might actually have the potential to block replication of the severe acute respiratory syndrome virus and through this mechanism might aid in protecting these vulnerable patients.[16]

To evaluate for B12 deficiency, clinicians should order a complete blood cell count and a serum B12, although screening individuals who are only considered to have an average risk of deficiency is not routinely recommended.[16] For replenishment patients usually receive parenteral therapy initially with a dose of 100 μg that begins as a daily treatment to eventually only requiring monthly treatment for the patient's lifetime.[6]

Vitamin C

In the United States, vitamin C deficiency ranks as the fourth most prevalent deficiency.[21] Vitamin C is an important player in immunologic health because it functions on a cellular level to signal neutrophils to the site of an active infection and to upregulate phagocytosis, which allows for the invading microbe to be killed.[21] Vitamin C is also a required component of collagen production.[22] In addition, there are vitamin C deposits in the skin, our first line of defense against invading microbes.[21] Vitamin C can be found in both the dermis and epidermis, although it is in great concentrations in the epidermis.[21]

The most extreme cases of vitamin C deficiency are in the form of scurvy. From a historical standpoint, scurvy was known for affecting sailors in ancient history due to the inability to store fresh foods including citrus products for long voyages. The body's natural storage of this vitamin is depleted in 1 to 3 months' time, and because humans cannot synthesize vitamin C, it must then be consumed to maintain healthy levels.[22,23]

The manifestations of early scurvy can often be missed because the complaints often are vague including malaise, fatigue, edema, and joint pain.[22,24] In pediatrics, it is estimated that 80% of scurvy cases have a musculoskeletal symptom at presentation with the knee being the most commonly affected joint in kids.[23] As scurvy continues to progress the symptoms get more catastrophic to gum ailments, loss of dentition, open wounds, ecchymosis, abnormal bleeding, and death.[22,24] The abnormal bleeding is thought to be associated to leaky vessels when collagen production is decreased without proper vitamin C levels; this complication can manifest itself with atraumatic hemarthrosis, petechia, purpura, and bleeding gums.[6,22] Scurvy is a clinical diagnosis but is additionally bolstered by a vitamin C/ascorbic acid serum assay that shows levels less than the normal range (45–90 μmol/L) or less than 0.2 mg/dL.[23,24] Replenishment is usually by way of oral supplements with doses ranging from 300 to 1000 mg every day.[6]

FAT SOLUBLE

The other category of vitamins includes those that are soluble in fat such as vitamins A, D, E, and K. These vitamins are stored within the tissues of the body and because of this are less easily washed out of the body, being stored for a longer period of time.[3]

Vitamin A

This vitamin has crucial properties on a cellular level to aid in epithelial cells differentiating throughout the body.[3] Vitamin A is absorbed into the body in the form of retinol; this primarily occurs in the small intestine.[25] The largest area of storage in the body for vitamin A is the liver.[9] Deficiency in vitamin A is perhaps best known for its association to blindness and is a preventable cause of blindness, particularly in lower-income countries.[6] An early manifestation of insufficient levels of vitamin A is night blindness[9,25]; this can be a crucial part of a patient's history to help uncover this nutritional issue.

Retinol deficiency can manifest as a variety of other ocular complications due to the changes of the eye's epithelium with patient possibly presenting with various complaints of dry eye, to local infections, to corneal ulcerations.[25,26] If left untreated, the integrity of the cornea continues to erode, and it will necrose and begin to soften, leading to perforation in a condition called keratomalacia.[25,26] On physical examination, one might find a pathognomonic characteristic called a Bitot spot.[27] Bitot spots are an accumulation on the cornea of white colored lesion that is often given the characteristic of a "foamy" consistency and that are easily identified on physical examination with only an ophthalmoscope.[25,27]

The WHO defines vitamin A deficiency as patient's serum level less than 0.70 μmol/L.[28] To adequately supplement the patient's vitamin A after confirming the diagnosis, treatment dosing can vary based on the severity, but a good starting range is 100,000 U orally every day for 3 days and then subsequently cutting the dose in half to 50,000 U every day orally for the next 2 weeks.[29]

Vitamin D

Inadequate amounts of vitamin D affect astronomical portions of the population with estimates that 1 billion individuals across the globe fall into this category.[30] Vitamin D is obtained in 2 pathways; one pathway involves synthesis by skin cells that are exposed to UV-B rays and the other path is by diet or supplements.[31] Given that sunlight is necessary for one pathway, this has been jeopardized with certain geographic limitations, urbanization, and increased sunscreen use.[6] In addition, the color of an individual's skin can affect synthesis because those with darker skin tones have higher levels of melanin pigment and are less capable of producing this vitamin by way of sunlight exposure.[32] Vitamin D exists in 2 forms D_2 and D_3, and the gold standard test to evaluate for deficiency is a serum test to evaluate for 25-hydroxyvitamin D levels. When these levels drop below 30 nmol/L an individual is considered to be deficient.[30,32] This deficiency is a prevalent issue with recent data showing that more than 90% of the US population is not ingesting the estimated average requirement of this vitamin.[32]

Vitamin D plays an important role in bone health by way of mineralization and is the most common cause of osteomalacia in adults.[6,31,33] In addition, there is association with calcium and phosphate in bone health; however, these minerals are outside of the scope of this article. Adults who are considered to be severely deficient and are therefore at risk for osteomalacia are often treated with a regimen that entails a loading dose 50,000 IU once a week for at least 2 months, although other regimens allow for this dose to be given 3 times a week for 1 month.[6,31] Children who are deficient in vitamin D present with rickets, a condition in which bone softening and deformities are present. To prevent rickets, 400 IU of vitamin D ingested daily is recommended.[33]

MINERALS

There are a variety of minerals that can play a part in nutritional deficiencies; for the scope of this article only iron is discussed because of the common nature of patients presenting with this deficiency.

Iron

Maintaining adequate iron levels in the body is a balancing act as 25 mg/d is required for cellular life and metabolism, but free iron can have a toxic effect on cells.[34] This goal of 25 mg iron each day is achieved in a variety of ways, including macrophages breaking down red blood cells and then harvesting their iron, using the body's iron storage, and by acquisition through an individual's diet. The storage of iron is distributed among several places in the body with the greatest areas of storage residing in the spleen, liver, and bone marrow.[34] An individual's diet should ideally consist of 1 to 2 mg consumption a day to balance the body's natural loss of about 1 to 2 mg/d, although this exact figure can be difficult to measure.[6,34]

Iron deficiency is the leading cause of anemia around the world.[6] Considering that approximately 27% of the population falls under the banner head of anemia, it is no small thing for iron deficiency to be the culprit.[34] Anemia is defined as hemoglobin levels less than 13 g/dL for men and less than 12 g/dL or nonpregnant women;

however, a normal hemoglobin level does not necessarily exclude this condition. Laboratory work to include serum ferritin will give the most accurate absolute value of iron in the body because it is a protein in the blood whose primary purpose is the storage of iron.[34] When considering ferritin levels, less than 30 ng/mL receives the label of low.[35] It is important to remember that ferritin values can be inaccurate in both the elderly and when there is an acute inflammation process occurring in the body because ferritin is an acute-phase reactant.[34] An acute-phase reactant is a marker of inflammation in the body that will have an altered serum level due to that inflammation.[36] Discovering that a patient has iron deficiency does not necessarily imply that this is a dietary issue alone because this deficiency can be caused by a multitude of causes, including inflammation, hemorrhage, or chronic diseases.

When deciding to replenish a patient's iron, there are a variety of options available with oral formulations being the most convenient and widely used. Oral supplementation is usually prescribed in a range of doses from 1 to 3 times a day, 100 to 200 mg for each dose.[35] An important side effect of this replenishment is to be aware that compliance is often an issue because as many as 70% of patients on this regimen report gastrointestinal (GI) side effects, which can be discouraging because 3 to 6 months of treatment is often required before the body's stores are replenished.[34,35] Intravenous iron is also available but is often saved for those individuals who are unable to complete oral supplementation or for patients in dire need of replenishment in a faster timetable than the months that are required in oral formulations.[34,35]

SPECIAL POPULATIONS

There are a variety of special populations that are at increased risk of exhibiting nutritionally deficiencies. The following sections will highlight a few of these populations.

Alcohol Use Disorder

Substance abuse is an ongoing epidemic in our world with estimates that alcohol use disorder (AUD) is third on the list of risk factors that end in disability or disease.[37] Individuals with AUD are notorious for being vulnerable to a large spectrum of nutritional deficiencies as well. In the United States, the primary form of liver disease is alcoholic cirrhosis with reports that anywhere from 20% to 90% of these patients have malnutrition.[2] Cirrhosis essentially causes the body to go into a state of accelerated starvation. The liver is additionally an important part of vitamin storage with 90% of the body's vitamin A residing there.[9] Patients with AUD are already predisposed to malnutrition, but then additionally the chronic ingestion of alcohol causes the body's stores of vitamin A to be repleted at a faster pace than in individuals who do not struggle with substance abuse. AUD additionally adds a layer of complexity to replenishing vitamin A in these patients because they can have hepatic toxicity that is caused by vitamin A.[9]

WE was discussed in the previous section on thiamine. Approximately 12.5% of alcoholics are thought to have WE.[8] It is often suspected that a large number of patients with WE or KS are actually missed clinically because approximately 80% to 85% of cases are only diagnosed postmortem.[7,8] To date, alcohol abuse is the most common cause of thiamine deficiency in our country.[6]

Previously discussed was pellagra, a disease related to niacin deficiency. There is another form of pellagra that can be seen in patients with AUD specifically in which aside from the typical findings of pellagra, patients can also present with an altered mental status.[9] This form can be problematic for the clinical picture and is often mistaken for alcohol intoxication, withdrawal, or another psychiatric pathology. This condition is then further complicated by the fact that replenishing certain B vitamins that are routinely supplemented in patients with AUD (B1, B6, and B12 of note) can then accelerate alcoholic pellagra.[9]

Down Syndrome

Down syndrome is a chromosomal abnormality that involves trisomy of chromosome 21. These patients have a variety of issues many of which link back to metabolic issues and nutritional complexities. Various studies have shown that patients with Down syndrome can be deficient in a variety of nutrients from the B vitamins, thiamine, iron, and vitamin A to name a few.[38] A large portion of pediatric patients who have Down syndrome have structural abnormalities of their GI tract ranging from pyloric stenosis to Hirschsprung to atresia of the GI tract.[39] In addition, these patients often have food preferences that are not conducive for balanced nutrition, opting for carbohydrate-rich foods and items that are easily chewed.[38] This preference of readily chewed food is supported by the fact that often these patients will have oral cavity complications like missing dentition, gum disease, or a large protruding tongue.[38,39]

Celiac Disease

Those affected with celiac disease (CD) have an immune response when exposed to food with gluten. When the body is introduced to gluten, it lodges an immune response that damages the villi of the small intestine perpetuating the issue of malabsorption as the villi surface area decreases.[6,40] Individuals with CD often additionally are inflicted with various forms of anemia from iron-deficient anemia to those resulting from deficiencies in B12 and B6.[41] In addition, these patients are at risk of being deficient in vitamin D, which can lead to issues maintaining healthy bones and putting individuals more at risk for conditions like that of osteomalacia and rickets.[40,41]

Status Post Bariatric Surgery

The prevalence of obesity continues to climb with estimates that as of 2016 approximately one-third of the population globally has a body mass index that categorizes them as overweight or obese.[42] As the population continues to gain in girth, the occurrence of bariatric procedures to treat this issue is also on the rise with as many as 500,000 procedures being performed around the world on an annual basis.[43] Obese patients tend to fall into 2 categories that dictate what type of procedure will be done; these 2 classifications are "volume eaters" who need a restrictive procedure or "sweet eaters" who require an intervention to change the absorption properties of their gut.[42,44] An example of a common restrictive procedure would be a lap band or sleeve gastrectomy, whereas the Roux-en-Y bypass is considered to be a combination of both restrictive and malabsorptive.[42] When looking at possible post–bariatric surgery issues, the malabsorptive procedures show a higher risk of nutritional deficiencies.[42]

Patients can have postoperative complications that can present themselves months to years after their actual procedure. It was found that anywhere from 30% to 49% of patients after undergoing either type of surgery were deficient in thiamine, presenting as far out as 6 months from their procedure.[42,44] Individuals who are thiamine deficient with characteristics of WE are often referred to as "bariatric beriberi."[43] The classic triad of symptoms was only seen in approximately 54% of the cases reviewed, which is considerably higher than what had been noted to manifest in patients with AUD.[8,43] A recent review of patients with bariatric beriberi showed that ataxia was the most prevalent finding followed by altered mental status and then the least common finding was eye movement abnormalities.[43]

Anemia is additionally a common issue for patients with post–bariatric procedure with 33% to 49% falling into the anemic category within the first 2 years after their surgery.[44] In healthy individuals for B12 to be absorbed, a substance called intrinsic factor must be available.[15] The parietal cells of the stomach are responsible for secreting intrinsic factor, and this allows for B12 to be absorbed later in the small intestine.[15] Patients who have had bariatric procedures done may have lower levels of intrinsic factor secreted, thus resulting in less absorption of B12 as just one aspect that makes them more susceptible to anemia.[15]

Elderly

With scientific advances in our modern world, people are simply living longer and there is an increase in the world's population of the elderly. It is estimated that between 2015 and 2030 the population of individuals 60 years or older will increase to a staggering 1.4 billion.[45] The elderly are disproportionately at risk for malnutrition, which means a large section of the population could be harmed by their lack of nutritional balance. It is estimated that 6% of the elderly living in out the community are affected and 39% of those that are hospitalized struggle with malnutrition.[46] A poor nutritional status has also been associated with frailty syndrome, which is considered to be an early stage of disability.[45] Thoughts as to why this special population is more affected than their younger cohorts range from medications, ill-fitting dentures, and changes in their attraction to food.[46]

The elderly can also be deficient in B12 with estimates that 15% to 20% of this population in the United States is deficient in B12.[15] One study demonstrated that vitamin D in inadequate amounts in the elderly could also be associated with long-term cognition issues.[47] This study looked at elderly patients who were seen for an acute illness in the emergency department who were at that evaluation found to be at their cognitive baseline; those who were deficient in vitamin D showed a worsening cognitive outcome 6 months down the road.[47] In addition, vitamin D plays a role in both bone health and muscle strength, and deficiencies in this can also play a role in an elderly patient's fall risk, which can cause significant morbidity and mortality for these patients.[30] Annually 300,000 patients are hospitalized due to injuries from falls that result in hip fractures alone.[48] Deficiencies in vitamin C have been linked to increased all-cause mortality in our older population as well.[21]

SUMMARY

Lack of proper nutritional can have devastating and even life-threatening consequences on an individual's state of health. Physician assistants have the ability to piece together a patient's history, physical examination, and laboratory test results to identify their potential nutritional weak spots and to treat for such; they can additionally serve as an advocate for special populations that have specific tendencies toward deficiency. Although the risks and outcomes differ, this is a global issue for which physician assistants can stand in the gap as a step toward balanced nutrition for their patients.

CLINICS CARE POINTS

- A helpful pneumonic to aid a practitioner in identifying which patient might be at risk is for WE is *WACO*: Wernicke ataxia, confusion, and ophthalmoplegia.[9]

- It is recommended that women of child-bearing status take 400 µg of folate daily to prevent detrimental neural tube birth defects.[13]

- Infants who are deficient in B12 often are breastfed by mothers who are deficient themselves or adhere to a vegan or vegetarian diet.[12]
- Bitot spots on an eye examination are pathognomonic for vitamin A deficiency.[27]

DISCLOSURE

The author has nothing to disclose.

REFERENCES

1. Darnton-Hill I. Public health aspects in the prevention and control of vitamin deficiencies. Curr Dev Nutr 2019;3(9):nzz075.
2. Dasarathy S. Nutrition and alcoholic liver disease: effects of alcoholism on nutrition, effects of nutrition on alcoholic liver disease, and nutritional therapies for alcoholic liver disease. Clin Liver Dis 2016;20(3):535–50.
3. Reddy P, Jialal I. Biochemistry, fat soluble vitamins. In: StatPearls. Treasure Island, FL: StatPearls Publishing; 2020.
4. Lykstad J, Sharma S. Biochemistry, Water Soluble Vitamins. In: StatPearls. Treasure Island, FL: StatPearls Publishing; 2020.
5. Shible AA, Ramadurai D, Gergen D, et al. Dry beriberi due to thiamine deficiency associated with peripheral neuropathy and Wernicke's Encephalopathy Mimicking Guillain-Barré syndrome: A case report and review of the literature. Am J Case Rep 2019;20:330–4.
6. Papadakis M, McPhee S. Current medical diagnosis and treatment. 57th edition. New York: McGraw-Hill Education; 2018.
7. Butterworth RF. Thiamin deficiency and brain disorders. Nutr Res Rev 2003;16(2): 277–84.
8. Donnino MW, Vega J, Miller J, et al. Myths and misconceptions of Wernicke's encephalopathy: what every emergency physician should know. Ann Emerg Med 2007;50(6):715–21.
9. Grock A, Lapoint J, Jhun P, Herbert M. Remember to take your vitamins. Ann Emerg Med 2016;68(3):389–91.
10. Paudel V, Chudal D. Classical pellagra, the disease of 4 Ds, the forgotten entity. Pan Afr Med J 2020;36:219.
11. Redzic S, Gupta V. Niacin Deficiency. In: StatPearls. Treasure Island, FL: StatPearls Publishing; 2020.
12. Black MM. Effects of vitamin B12 and folate deficiency on brain development in children. Food Nutr Bull 2008;29(2 Suppl):S126–31.
13. Folic Acid. Centers for Disease Control and Prevention. Available at: https://www.cdc.gov/ncbddd/folicacid/index.html. Accessed February 28, 2021.
14. Czeizel AE, Dudás I, Vereczkey A, et al. Folate deficiency and folic acid supplementation: the prevention of neural-tube defects and congenital heart defects. Nutrients 2013;5(11):4760–75.
15. Hannibal L, Lysne V, Bjørke-Monsen AL, et al. Biomarkers and algorithms for the diagnosis of vitamin B12 deficiency [published correction appears in Front Mol Biosci. 2017 Aug 08;4:53]. Front Mol Biosci 2016;3:27.
16. Langan RC, Goodbred AJ. Vitamin B12 Deficiency: Recognition and Management. Am Fam Physician 2017;96(6):384–9.
17. Aguirre JA, Donato ML, Buscio M, et al. Compromiso neurológico grave por déficit de vitamina B12 en lactantes hijos de madres veganas y vegetarianas

[Serious neurological compromise due to vitamin B12 deficiency in infants of vegan and vegetarian mothers]. Arch Argent Pediatr 2019;117(4):e420–4.

18. Bousselamti A, El Hasbaoui B, Echahdi H, et al. Psychomotor regression due to vitamin B12 deficiency. Pan Afr Med J 2018;30:152.

19. Wee AKH. COVID-19's toll on the elderly and those with diabetes mellitus - Is vitamin B12 deficiency an accomplice? Med Hypotheses 2021;146:110374.

20. Ahmed MA. Metformin and vitamin B12 deficiency: Where do we stand? J Pharm Pharm Sci 2016;19(3):382–98.

21. Carr AC, Maggini S. Vitamin C and immune function. Nutrients 2017;9(11):1211.

22. Wijkmans RA, Talsma K. Modern scurvy. J Surg Case Rep 2016;2016(1):rjv168.

23. Miraj F, Abdullah A. Scurvy: Forgotten diagnosis, but still exist. Int J Surg Case Rep 2020;68:263–6.

24. Gordon BL, Galati J, Yang S, et al. Vitamin C deficiency: an under-recognized condition in crohn's disease. ACG Case Rep J 2020;7(7):e00424.

25. Cheshire J, Kolli S. Vitamin A deficiency due to chronic malabsorption: an ophthalmic manifestation of a systemic condition [published correction appears in BMJ Case Rep. 2017 Aug 28;2017:]. BMJ Case Rep 2017;2017. bcr2017220024.

26. Kopecký A, Benda F, Němčanský J. Xerosis in Patient with vitamin A deficiency - a Case Report. Xeróza u pacientky s deficiencí vitaminu A. Cesk Slov Oftalmol 2018;73(5–6):222–4.

27. Sahile Z, Yilma D, Tezera R, et al. Prevalence of vitamin A deficiency among pre-school children in Ethiopia: a systematic review and meta-analysis. Biomed Res Int 2020;202:8032894.

28. World Health Organization. Vitamin A supplementation. 2021. Available at: https://www.who.int/elena/titles/full_recommendations/vitamina_supp/en/. [Accessed 14 February 2021].

29. Vitamin A (retinol) Adult Dosing - Epocrates Online. Online.epocrates.com. 2021. Available at: https://online.epocrates.com/u/1014054/vitamin%20A%20(retinol)/Adult%20Dosing. [Accessed 23 February 2021].

30. Sahota O. Understanding vitamin D deficiency. Age Ageing 2014;43(5):589–91.

31. Kennel KA, Drake MT, Hurley DL. Vitamin D deficiency in adults: when to test and how to treat. Mayo Clin Proc 2010;85(8):752–8.

32. Office of Dietary Supplements - Vitamin D. Ods.od.nih.gov. Available at: https://ods.od.nih.gov/factsheets/VitaminD-HealthProfessional/#h5. Accessed February 27, 2021.

33. Bouillon R, Marcocci C, Carmeliet G, et al. Skeletal and Extraskeletal Actions of Vitamin D: current evidence and outstanding questions. Endocr Rev 2019;40(4):1109–51.

34. Ning S, Zeller MP. Management of iron deficiency. Hematol Am Soc Hematol Educ Program 2019;2019(1):315–22.

35. Muñoz M, Gómez-Ramírez S, Besser M, et al. Current misconceptions in diagnosis and management of iron deficiency. Blood Transfus 2017;15(5):422–37.

36. Gulhar R, Ashraf MA, Jialal I. Physiology, acute phase reactants. In: StatPearls. Treasure Island, FL: StatPearls Publishing; 2020.

37. Rocco A, Compare D, Angrisani D, et al. Alcoholic disease: liver and beyond. World J Gastroenterol 2014;20(40):14652–9.

38. Mazurek D, Wyka J. Down syndrome–genetic and nutritional aspects of accompanying disorders. Rocz Panstw Zakl Hig 2015;66(3):189–94.

39. Newton RW, Puri S, Marder L. Down syndrome: current perspectives. Mac Keith Press. 2015. Available at: http://search.ebscohost.com.ezproxy.hsutx.edu:2048/

login.aspx?direct=true&db=e000xna&AN=975726&site=eds-live&scope=site. [Accessed 28 February 2021].

40. Garner P. Celiac disease : risk factors, health implications and dietary management. Nova Science Publishers, Inc. 2016. Available at: http://search.ebscohost.com.ezproxy.hsutx.edu:2048/login.aspx?direct=true&db=e000xna&AN=1406245&site=eds-live&scope=site. [Accessed 28 February 2021].

41. Kreutz JM, Adriaanse MPM, van der Ploeg EMC, et al. Narrative review: nutrient deficiencies in adults and children with treated and untreated celiac disease. Nutrients 2020;12(2):500.

42. Mesureur L, Arvanitakis M. Metabolic and nutritional complications of bariatric surgery: a review. Acta Gastroenterol Belg 2017;80(4):515–25.

43. Oudman E, Wijnia JW, van Dam M, et al. Preventing Wernicke encephalopathy after bariatric surgery. Obes Surg 2018;28(7):2060–8.

44. Lupoli R, Lembo E, Saldalamacchia G, et al. Bariatric surgery and long-term nutritional issues. World J Diabetes 2017;8(11):464–74.

45. Lorenzo-López L, Maseda A, de Labra C, et al. Nutritional determinants of frailty in older adults: A systematic review. BMC Geriatr 2017;17(1):108.

46. Pereira GF, Bulik CM, Weaver MA, et al. Malnutrition among cognitively intact, noncritically ill older adults in the emergency department. Ann Emerg Med 2015;65(1):85–91.

47. Evans CS, Self W, Ginde AA, et al. Vitamin D deficiency and long-term cognitive impairment among older adult emergency department patients. West J Emerg Med 2019;20(6):926–30.

48. Important Facts about Falls | Home and Recreational Safety | CDC Injury Center. Cdc.gov. Available at: https://www.cdc.gov/homeandrecreationalsafety/falls/adultfalls.html. Accessed February 28, 2021.

Eosinophilic Esophagitis
An Emerging Disorder for Co-management

Kathy J. Robinson, DHSc, MPAS, PA-C*

KEYWORDS

- Eosinophilic esophagitis • Eosinophilic esophagitis diagnosis
- Eosinophilic esophagitis treatment

KEY POINTS

- Eosinophilic esophagitis is a cause of dysphagia and food impaction in children and adults.
- Diagnosis is made based on clinical presentation and esophageal biopsy.
- Disease management is long term and includes treatment modalities, including proton pump inhibitor therapy, swallowed topical steroids, elimination diet, and dilation of esophageal strictures with the goal of illness remission.
- Physician assistants play a crucial role in identifying, diagnosing, and providing referral, care coordination, symptom management, and patient education in primary care and specialty care settings.

INTRODUCTION

The esophagus is the muscular tube that connects the pharynx with the stomach and allows passage of food through the upper esophageal sphincter into the stomach for digestion. The esophagus plays a role in the gastrointestinal (GI) and immunologic systems. If the esophageal mucosa is healthy, the passage of food is effortless for the patient. The mouth and esophagus are among the first immunologic defenders in the human body, and under normal physiologic conditions, they are devoid of eosinophils.[1] The esophageal mucosa defends the human body using mucus, bicarbonate, defensins, lymphocytes, leukocytes, mast cells, and squamous epithelial cells.[2] Normal esophageal mucosa, unlike the rest of the GI tract, does not include the presence of eosinophils.[2] The pathology of eosinophilic esophagitis (EoE) can change the normal function of the esophagus, make the patients aware of solid food descending, cause them to experience dysphagia,[2] and put them at risk of food impaction, among other complications. Over time, the eosinophils infiltrate the esophageal epithelium, which may lead to esophageal stenosis and fibrosis.[3]

Hardin-Simmons University, 2200 Hickory Street, HSU Box 16236, Abilene, TX 79698, USA
* Corresponding author.
E-mail address: Kathy.robinson@hsutx.edu

Physician Assist Clin 6 (2021) 593–602
https://doi.org/10.1016/j.cpha.2021.05.004
2405-7991/21/© 2021 Elsevier Inc. All rights reserved.

History

Landres and colleagues first reported EoE in 1978, and Attwood and colleagues recognized EoE as a distinct clinical condition in 1993.[1] EoE is becoming increasingly recognized in pediatric and adult populations and requires comanagement with multiple specialists, including allergist/immunologists, gastroenterologists, and otolaryngologists. Pathologists and dieticians are also part of the interprofessional team needed to help patients with disease remission and management of symptoms. A high degree of suspicion for EoE may lead to earlier diagnosis and better treatment outcomes for all patient populations. **Table 1** has a list of common abbreviations related to this disorder.

BACKGROUND
Eosinophilic Esophagitis and Atopic Disease

Patients with a diagnosis of EoE often have an atopic disease, including asthma, allergic rhinitis, atopic dermatitis, immunoglobulin E (IgE)-mediated food allergy, and pollen-food allergy syndrome (PFAS). Letner and colleagues indicate that there are limited data to correlate PFAS with EoE.[3] PFAS syndrome may also be referred to as oral allergy syndrome (OAS), which produces an IgE-mediated hypersensitivity reaction having symptoms based on cross-reactivity of environmental allergens and food allergens.[3] Further studies are underway to increase understanding of the similarities and differences between PFAS and EoE.[3] Care coordination for patients with EoE is essential for allergy/immunologists to consider treating and evaluating comorbid atopic diseases.

Eosinophilic Esophagitis Versus Gastroesophageal Reflux Disease

Clinical presentation of EoE can overlap with signs and symptoms of gastroesophageal reflux disease (GERD), especially in the adult population.[4] GERD and EoE are the first and second most common causes, respectively, of esophagitis and esophageal dysfunction.[4] The diagnosis of EoE requires a biopsy with the presence of more than 15 eosinophils per high-powered field (HPF) in one or more esophageal biopsies.[1] Also, diagnosis of EoE includes a normal pH.[1] The nuanced clinical presentation between EoE and GERD can be differentiated by a history of heartburn and regurgitation for patients with GERD and solid food dysphagia and food impaction in patients with EoE.[2] GERD is primarily characterized as a chronic mucosal inflammation disease,

Table 1 Topic abbreviations	
Abbreviation	**Term**
EoE	Eosinophilic esophagitis
Eos/hpf	Eosinophils/high-powered field
PPI	Proton pump inhibitor
MDI	Metered-dose inhaler
EREFS	Eosinophilic esophagitis endoscopic reference score
FED	Food elimination diet
ICS	Topical corticosteroids
ECP	Eosinophilic cationic protein
PFAS	Pollen-food allergy syndrome
GERD	Gastroesophageal reflux disease
IBD	Inflammatory bowel disorder

and in the worst cases, a disease of destructive esophageal tissue remodeling.[2] Clinical symptoms of GERD and EoE continue to have overlapping characteristics, so further endoscopic, allergic, and pathologic studies are needed to confirm the EoE diagnosis.

DISCUSSION
Clinical Presentation

Patients diagnosed with EoE often experience dysphagia for solid foods, frequent food impaction,[5] and noncardiac chest pain.[1] Adult patients may compensate for symptoms by eating slowly, cutting food into smaller pieces, excessive chewing, and frequent drinking during extended mealtimes.[2] GERD-like symptoms have also been reported in about one-third of patients with a diagnosis of EoE.[5] Pediatric patients may present with vomiting, regurgitation, heartburn, and in some cases, failure to thrive.[6] Parents of infants and toddlers with EoE may report difficulty in feeding, choking, and food refusal.[2,6] Physician assistants (PAs) working in clinical setting with pediatric populations should track the infant's/child's progress on the growth chart and listen carefully to the parent if he or she expresses distress about the infant's/child's behavior during or after feeding.

Diagnosis

EoE is characterized by esophageal inflammation, and diagnosis requires at least 15 eosinophils per HPF on esophageal biopsies.[6] The presence of eosinophils per HPF may vary based on the site and the biopsy specimen.[7] Two or more biopsies are recommended and should be obtained from the proximal and distal esophagus.[1] The eosinophil count is not the sole foundation of the disease. The clinical presentation should also be considered when making a diagnosis. An interdisciplinary approach is ideal for the care of patients with EoE. Referrals should be timely with supporting documentation.

Differential Diagnosis

To diagnose EoE, the patient should be referred to an allergy/immunologist and gastroenterologist. Differential diagnoses that should be ruled out include GERD, achalasia, esophageal cancer, hypereosinophilic syndrome, infection, Crohn disease, and drug allergies.[2] Other disorders may accompany EoE and must be considered: eosinophilic gastroenteritis, parasitic and fungal infections, inflammatory bowel disorders, hypereosinophilic syndrome, and esophageal leiomyomatosis, myeloproliferative disorders, allergic vasculitis, and scleroderma.[1] EoE differs in clinical presentation PFAS, also known as OAS. PFAS presents with oral pharyngeal pruritis, angioedema, oral pruritis/itching, and tingling soon after eating the trigger food.[3] The patient symptoms in PFAS appear within minutes of trigger food ingestion and result from sensitization and cross-reactivity of food and aeroallergens.[3]

Causes of esophageal eosinophilia may include eosinophilic gastroenteritis, celiac disease, Crohn disease, hypereosinophilic syndrome, achalasia, hypersensitivity to drugs, vasculitis, pemphigus, or connective tissue disease.[8]

It is important to note that the patient's self-reported dysphagia symptoms may originate from multiple origins and causes. Medical providers should keep a broad differential diagnosis in mind. Dysphagia can arise from pathology in the oropharyngeal, esophageal, and gastric areas and may be mechanical, neuromuscular, or inflammatory in nature.[9] Consensus panel recommendations emphasize that manifestations or pathologic data should not be interpreted in isolation for patients with EoE.[10]

SUMMARY

A diagnosis of EoE for a patient presents a potential decrease in quality of life for a patient of any age. PAs are key clinicians for diagnosis, treatment, referral to specialty care, and care coordination. PAs should keep a high level of suspicion for a diagnosis of EoE in a pediatric or adult patient who presents with dysphagia and feeding and eating concerns. Many of the presenting signs and symptoms mimic those of gastroesophageal reflux and may lead to delayed diagnosis. Delayed diagnosis may lead to esophageal strictures and narrowing of the esophageal lumen.[6]

NATURE OF THE PROBLEM
Patient Quality of Life

Pediatric and adult symptoms of EoE can significantly affect patient and caregiver quality of life. Many patients suffer from the embarrassment that feeding and eating habits create at home and social settings. Patients may develop coping mechanisms in response to symptoms such as avoiding highly textured foods that are difficult to swallow and increased intake of liquids during mealtimes.[2] Behavioral coping mechanisms during mealtime can significantly affect social interactions for patients diagnosed with EoE.

In the case that EoE diagnosis is delayed, the patient might present with food impaction, esophageal stenosis, a history of symptoms that become progressively worse, and eosinophilic infiltration of the esophagus that is confirmed by biopsy.[11] A delayed diagnosis may put the patient at risk for esophageal rupture because of an unidentified diagnosis.[11] EoE is not associated with a higher risk of malignancy, but the associated symptoms affect the patient quality of life.[12] Goals for treatment of EoE should include symptom reduction, histologic remission of the disease, reduction of esophageal remodeling and formation of strictures, and improvement of patient quality of life.[12]

OBSERVATION/ASSESSMENT/EVALUATION
Dysphagia and Feeding Screening Questionnaires

In addition to a complete history and physical examination, there are several instruments used assess the difficulties patients may be having with dysphagia and feeding problems.[12] For children, the Pediatric EoE Symptom Score (PEESSv2.) gathers information about patient symptoms in the area of dysphagia, GERD, nausea/vomiting, and pain.[12] For the adult patient populations, symptom screening tools include the EoE Activity Index (EEsAI) and the Dysphagia Symptom Questionnaire.[12] The EEsAI gauges difficulties the patient feels he or she will encounter with different food consistencies and behavioral modifications for the food consistencies.[12] The Dysphagia Symptom Questionnaire is a shorter 3-item electronic diary that helps patients record when they have dysphagia symptoms and days they avoid solid foods.[12] Dysphagia and feeding screening questionnaires are important data collection tools than can be used to track patient symptoms to support a referral for a specialist evaluation.

Eosinophilic Esophagitis Endoscopic Reference Score

Eosinophilic esophagitis Endoscopic Reference Score (EREFS) can guide the recognition and reporting of primary endoscopic findings in patients with EoE.[13] The EREFS rates 5 endoscopic findings as none, mild, moderate, and severe.[13] The preliminary endoscopic findings in EoE are the presence of rings, exudates, furrows, edemas, and strictures.[13] The EREFS defines the specific grading of rings based on the ability of standard diagnostic endoscope to pass through the diameter of the esophagus.[13] The lesions are graded based on the percentage of the esophageal surface involvement.[13]

PREVALENCE/INCIDENCE AND MORTALITY RATES

Eosinophilic esophagitis was reported in the literature as an allergic disease in 1995. Since that time, the prevalence has increased, with the estimated pooled prevalence of 56.7 cases per 100,000 people in the United States.[11] Males and individuals of Caucasian race are more likely to have a diagnosis of EoE.[4] The increased incidence in males and those of Caucasian race is not understood at this time. There seems to be a genetic predisposition for risk factors such as gut barrier function, oral antigen or aeroallergen exposure, and microbiome impairment.[4] A patient diagnosed with EoE is often diagnosed with allergic diseases, including food allergy, asthma, eczema, and/or allergic rhinitis.[4] A diagnosis of EoE can occur at any age, with various symptom constellations; however, symptoms generally begin in childhood. Actual age varies on the infant's or child's ability to report symptoms.[4]

GOALS

The goals of therapy for EoE in patients of all ages include resolving symptoms and achieving and maintaining remission of the disease based on reducing eosinophilic mucosal inflammation.[12] Additional goals for treatment include preventing esophageal fibrosis and food impaction, monitoring and mitigating adverse effects of medications, and minimizing nutritional deficiencies associated with feeding and eating problems.[12] All the goals combined add to an improved quality of life for patients with a diagnosis of EoE.

EVALUATION

There is a connection between EoE and atopy, so it is useful to determine the patient's sensitivity to environmental allergens and aeroallergens and food sensitivity.[4] Positive results for patients with EoE are common when skin prick testing and atopy patch testing are conducted for foods and/or aeroallergens.[14] Skin prick testing and atopy patch testing may be useful to assess the patient's overall atopy profile. Appropriate treatment of atopic diseases may improve the overall quality of life for patients diagnosed with EoE.

NEWEST GUIDELINES

Therapeutic and treatment guidelines for EoE were first published in 2007, followed by an update in 2011. Guideline recommendations by pediatric gastroenterologists were published in 2011 under the acronym ESPGHAN (European Society for Pediatric Gastroenterology, Hepatology and Nutrition).[5] Additional guidelines were published internationally in 2017 based on the GRADE (Grading of Recommendations Assessment, Development, and Evaluation) methodology.[5] The 2017 guidelines recognize that treatment with a proton pump inhibitor (PPI), swallowed inhaled corticosteroids, or elimination diets may improve clinical symptoms and histologic findings.[5] Swallowed inhaled corticosteroids are often prescribed for the treatment of EoE in the form of fluticasone meter dose inhaler. The patient is instructed to remove the cap of the inhaler, hold the inhaler with the mouthpiece at the bottom, and shake as recommended by the manufacturer. After the mouthpiece is inserted into the mouth, the patient is instructed to press the inhaler and swallow without breathing until swallowing is complete. The patient should not eat or drink for 30 minutes after the dose is administered. The inhaled corticosteroid is deposited on the patient's esophageal lining instead of being inhaled into the lungs.

In June 2020, David Johnson, professor of medicine and chief of gastroenterology at Eastern Virginia Medical School in Norfolk, Virginia, gave an update on Medscape summarizing the new EoE guidelines.[15] His article and recorded message were titled New Eosinophilic Esophagitis Guidelines: What You Need to Know." The new guidelines have been published by the American Gastroenterological Association Institute and the Joint Task Force on Allergy-Immunology Practice Parameters. The updated guidelines included a technical review explaining how the recommendations were formulated.[15] Johnson summarized the definition of remission, weighting the value of PPIs, glucocorticosteroids, esophageal dilation, endoscopic evaluation, medical therapy, and emerging therapies.[15]

Defining Remission

The guidelines define treatment effect by failing to achieve histologic remission of less than 15 eosinophils per high-powered filed as the gold standard.[15] Repeat esophageal biopsies are required to track disease progression, treatment outcomes, and to determine if the patient's disease is in remission.

Use of Proton Pump Inhibitors

The updated guidelines removed a PPI trial from the diagnostic criteria for EoE. The guidelines confirm recommend use of PPIs as a treatment modality, although Johnson noted that the use is conditional given the overall evidence and the lack of prospective studies.[15]

Glucocorticosteroids

Johnson noted that glucocorticosteroids have been studied extensively in topical and systemic form.[15] Fluticasone has been found efficacious, whether the esophageal delivery is by inhalation or swallowing.[15]

Swallowed Topical Steroids

Off-label use of swallowed inhaled topical steroids has long been the mainstay of treatment for EoE.[16] The use of viscous budesonide allows for deposition on the esophageal epithelial area and helps restore the barrier function of the esophagus to prevent remodeling.[16] Both budesonide and fluticasone propionate were significantly superior to placebo in decreasing the eosinophil density in the esophageal mucosa.[12] Instruction and patient education are essential to make sure that the swallowed inhaled corticosteroid is deposited on the esophageal lining instead of inhaled per the usual manufacturer instructions. Instruction should include the use of the meter dose inhaler per the manufacturer's instructions, with the modification that the patient should press the inhaler, and then swallow. The patient should not breathe until the medicine is swallowed.

Viscous budesonide exposes the esophageal epithelium to the medication longer than the nebulized form of budesonide.[16] Swallowed topical corticosteroids have a more favorable safety profile than systemic corticosteroid use.[12] About 10% of patients in all age groups suffer from esophageal candidiasis using swallowed topical corticosteroids.[12] It is important to note that swallowed topical corticosteroids do not require a corticosteroid withdrawal when compared with long-term systemic corticosteroid use.[12] Treatment with systemic corticosteroids is not indicated in the treatment of EoE.[12] Patient medication adherence remains a barrier to long-term treatment with swallowed topical corticosteroids[16]

Elemental Diets

The new guidelines specifically recommend the 6-food elimination diet. However, it is noted that the 8-food elimination diet can be used and includes peanuts and tree nuts and finned fish and shellfish.[15] The author recommends that consultation with a dietician be considered. The new guidelines recommend eliminating the 2 most common foods first as part of an overall food elimination diet.[15] Recommendations specifically state that the first foods to be eliminated should be wheat and milk.[15]

Esophageal Dilatation

The guidelines indicate that dilation is helpful for adults with EOE who have dysphagia caused by a stricture.[15] Patients requiring esophageal dilatation must be referred to a gastroenterologist for the procedure. Care coordination can be facilitated by a primary care PA.

Emerging Therapies

There are several new treatment approaches discussed in the guidelines, including interleukin (IL)-4, 5, and 13, and several immunomodulators and eosinophil release inhibitors.[15] It should be highlighted that the guidelines only recommend these treatments if used in the context of a clinical study.[15]

APPLICATION
Referrals and Coordination of Care

A PA evaluating a patient with symptoms of EoE should keep an open differential diagnosis and obtain a complete history and perform a complete physical examination to assess the patient. Specialist referral and care coordination are fundamental for the PA to consider if the patient is identified in a primary care setting. The diagnostic reports, consultation notes, and treatment recommendations will be returned to the primary care provider after evaluation. After all information is reviewed, the primary care provider can begin follow-up and coordination of referrals and provide patient education as needed.

Once a patient is identified with a possible diagnosis of EoE, he or she should be referred to a gastroenterology team and allergist for coordination of care. If the specialist recommends a food elimination diet, the patient should be referred to a dietician for care coordination.

THERAPEUTIC OPTIONS

EoE is a chronic disorder that requires long-term treatment. Therapeutic approaches include PPIs, swallowed topical steroids, dietary restriction, and endoscopic dilation.[17] If continuous therapy is discontinued, patients will experience a return of clinical symptoms.

Proton Pump Inhibitors

PPIs are often a therapeutic option before or after the diagnosis of EoE. About one-third of patients with clinical and endoscopic evidence of EoE will respond to monotherapy with PPIs.[4] EoE that responds to PPI monotherapy is referred to as PPI-responsive esophageal eosinophilia (PPI-REE).

The 2017 EoE guidelines recommend that PPIs be considered the first line treatment for patients with esophageal disfunction symptoms and have esophageal eosinophilia as evidenced on biopsy.[17] According to the most recent guidelines, treatment with PPI is conditional, and a trial of PPIs has been removed from the diagnostic criteria.[15]

Dietary Restriction

The goal of dietary restriction in patients with EoE includes identification of the trigger foods for the patient.[12] Food elimination diets identify the food trigger as the primary goal with the secondary goals of reducing symptoms and disease complications and decreasing the histologic reference point.[12]

Multiple studies support the role of food elimination diets in the treatment of the disease. Food elimination diets of the strictest type eliminate 6 foods. The 6-food elimination diet (SFED) has the patient abstain from eating wheat, dairy, egg, soy, peanuts/tree nuts, and fish/shellfish.[3] Evidence suggests that between 90% of children and 75% of adults experience disease remission when placed on a food elimination diet.[3] Outcomes for symptom reduction are influenced by patient adherence to a food elimination diet and the duration of abstinence from the foods. Food elimination diet effects may be less than expected if processed/prepared foods are contaminated with restricted foods and may be ingested unknowingly by the patient.[8] Some studies indicate that up to one-third of patients do not realize a reduction in symptoms with food elimination diet.[3] When foods are reintroduced after an elimination diet, cow's milk was most involved in the development of EoE for children and adults.[8] The food elimination diet is still considered an option as an empiric treatment of EoE, and the role of environmental or aeroallergens is yet to be determined and should not be underestimated. Drawbacks or barriers to elimination diets include decreased patient compliance, patient weight loss, if not consuming adequate calories, and the high cost of a modified diet.[18] Patient food preference and taste remain barriers to maintenance of a food elimination diet.

Endoscopic Dilation

Endoscopic features that may be present in patients with EoE include linear furrowing, concentric rings, whitish vesicles scattered over the mucosal surface, Schatzki ring, small-caliber esophagus, linear superficial mucosal tears, and esophageal ulcers and/or strictures.[14] Esophageal dilatation may be required for patients with severe symptoms. A specialist should be consulted for evaluation and to determine the dilatation technique based on the patient's age, the severity of strictures, and other clinical features.[4]

CONTROVERSIES

Coordination of care is critical in the treatment of patients with EoE. With the treatment modalities available, the application of more than 1 treatment at a time may make it difficult to discern which treatment is most effective for controlling symptoms.[12] Without knowing exactly which intervention is creating the change in symptoms, it is difficult to maintain that intervention long term.[12]

However, the literature demonstrates combing therapy for patients is beneficial for symptom relief.[6] PAs involved in the care of patients with EoE should seek to refer and treat patients based on the newest guidelines and evidence base. Controversy remains about the approach and timing of treatment, and this may be affected by a delay of diagnosis and access to specialty care for some patients.

EPIDEMIOLOGY

EoE affects men of the white race predominantly, and there is evidence of family aggregation.[8] The epidemiology of EoE has a basis in both environmental and genetic factors.[8] EoE is associated with atopic disease and IgE-mediated food allergies and affects both children and adults.[8] Barrier dysfunction and T-helper 2 cell inflammation play a role in the development of the disease.[8] Histologic evidence of disease may not correlate with symptoms of the disease.[8]

FUTURE DIRECTIONS

Exciting new treatments for patients with EoE are under development. Currently, there are several biologic therapies under investigation, as well as budesonide effervescent tablets. The budesonide tablets have recently been approved in Europe.[16]

Biologics used for TH2-mediated disease have entered phase II and phase III trials in patients with EoE.[16] Biologic agents targeting cytokines, including IL-4, IL-5, and IL-13, have been studied.[16] Additionally, studies are investigating biologic agents targeting IgE and tumor necrosis factor in patients with a diagnosis if EoE.[16]

Monoclonal antibodies directed at specific cytokines indicated in EoE are currently under evaluation.[5] Reslizumab has been studied in children and adolescents with EoE.[19] Reslizumab used to inhibit IL-5 resulted in the reduction of eosinophil counts in patients with EoE.[19] The changes in eosinophil histology and clinical symptoms remain unclear.[19]

As new treatment modalities develop, there is a growing need to identify noninvasive histologic markers that may diagnose and monitor disease procession and treatment.[8] At this time, repeat esophageal biopsies are needed to diagnose and monitor the disease progression.

SUMMARY

EoE is a chronic immune- and antigen-mediated esophageal disease. The disease presents at any age with dysphagia and possibly food impaction. Early detection of the disease and referral for comanagement dramatically improve patient outcomes and quality of life. Comanagement is multidisciplinary, and PAs play a key role in recognizing the illness by keeping EoE on the differential diagnosis and making timely referrals for evaluation.

CLINICS CARE POINTS

- The patient care team should include primary care providers, pediatricians, allergists/immunologists, gastroenterologists, otolaryngologists, pathologists, dieticians, and epidemiologists.[5]

- Patient and family history of atopy, as well as allergy assessment, may yield important clues and lead to timely diagnosis of EoE.

- Diagnosis is based on the patient's clinical presentation, esophageal biopsies, and histologic findings.[1]

- Medical and surgical management must be considered for the best patient outcomes.[11]

- The US Food and Drug Administration has not approved a single agent for the treatment of EoE.[16]

- Off-label use of swallowed topical corticosteroids, dietary restriction, and endoscopic dilation are the current treatment modalities.[16]

- Treatment strategies include pharmacologic therapy, avoidance of trigger foods, food elimination diets, pharmacologic treatment, and mechanical dilations of the esophagus when and if needed.[4]

- Signs and symptoms may mimic GERD.

DISCLOSURE STATEMENT

The author has nothing to disclose.

REFERENCES

1. Khalil MM, Patrwary MRI, Miah MR, et al. Eosinophilic esophagitis: An increasingly recognized disease in recent era. J Med 2019;20(2):109–11.
2. Inage E, Furuta GT, Menard-Katcher C, et al. Eosinophilic esophagitis: pathophysiology and its clinical implications. Am J Physiol Garointertest Liver Physiol 2018;315:G879–86.
3. Letner D, Farris A, Khalili H, et al. Pollen-food allergy syndrome is a common allergic comorbidity in adults with eosinophilic esophagitis. Dis Esophagus 2017;31:1–8.
4. Iuliano S, Minelli R, Vincenzi, et al. Eosinophilic esophagitis in pediatric age, state of the art and review of literature. Acta Biomed 2018;89(8):20–6.
5. Schoepfer A, Blanchard C, Dawson H, et al. Eosinophilic esophagitis: Latest insights from diagnosis to therapy. Ann N.Y Acad Sci 2018;84–93.
6. Reed CC, Safta AM, Qasem S, et al. Combined and alternating topical steroids and food elimination diet for the treatment of eosinophilic esophagitis. Dig Dis Sci 2018;63:2381–8.
7. Kim GH, Park YS, Jung KW, et al. An increasing trend of eosinophilic esophagitis in Korea and the clinical implication of the biomarkers to determine disease activity and treatment response in eosinophilic esophagitis. J Neurogastroenterol Motil 2019;25(4):525–33.
8. Torrijos EG, Gonzalez-Mendiola R, Alvarado M, et al. Eosinophilic esophagitis: review and update. Front Med 2018;5(247):1–15.
9. Kumar K, Makker J, Tariq H, et al. Co-occurrence of rarest type of dysphagia Lusoria (Type N-1) and eosinophilic esophagitis in a cognitively disabled individual. Case Rep Med 2019;2019(ID2890635):1–6.
10. Lucendo AJ, Molina-Infante J, Arias A, et al. Guidelines on eosinophilic esophagitis: evience-based statements and recommendations for diagnosis and management in children and adults. United Eur Gastroenterol J 2017;5(3):335–58.
11. Issa D, Alwatari Y, Smallfield G, et al. Spontaneous transmural perforation in eosinophilic esophagitis: RARE case presentation and role of esophageal stenting. J Surg Case Rep 2019;6:1–3.
12. Munoz-Persy M, Lucendo A. Treatment of eosinophilic esophagitis in the pediatric patient: an evidence-based approach. Eur J Pediatr 2018;117:649–63.
13. Cengiz C. Serum eosinophilic cationic protein is correlated with food impaction and endoscopic severity in eosinophilic esophagitis. Turk J Gastroenterol 2019; 30(4):345–9.
14. Carr S, Chan E, Watson W. Eosinophilic esophagitis. Allergy Asthma Clin Immunol 2018;14(Suppl 2):58.
15. Johnson DA. New eosinophilic esophagitis guidelines: what you need to know. Medscape. 2020. Available at: www.medscape.com. Accessed September 9, 2020.
16. Greuter T, Hirano I, Dellon E. Emerging therapies for eosinophilic esophagitis. J Allergy Clin Immunol 2020;145(1):38–45.
17. Ferreira CT, Vieira MC, Furuta GT, et al. Eosinophilic esophagitis – Where are we today? J Pediatr 2019;95(3):275–81.
18. Casiraghi A, Gennari CG, Musazzi UM. Mucoadhesive budesonide formulation for the treatment of eosinophilic esophagitis. Pharmaceutics 2020;12(211):1–12.
19. Spergel JM, Rothenberg ME, Collins MH, et al. Reslizumab in children and adolescents with eosinophilic esophagitis: results of a double-blind, randomized, placebo-controlled trial. J Allergy Clin Immunol 2012;129(2):456–63.e3.

Pathophysiology of Peptic Ulcer Disease

Elisabeth J. Shell, MPAS, PhD, PA-C

KEYWORDS

- PUD • *H pylori* • Virulence factors • Immune evasion
- Nonsteroidal antiinflammatory drugs

KEY POINTS

- Peptic ulcer disease (PUD) consists of 2 types of ulcers, gastric and duodenal ulcers.
- The 2 primary causes of PUD are mediated by the pathogen, *Helicobacter pylori*, and by nonsteroidal antiinflammatory drugs.
- *H pylori* has an arsenal of virulence factors that aid in colonization and persistence in the unfavorable environment to the stomach.
- *H pylori* also hijacks and evades host immune responses.
- Nonsteroidal antiinflammatory drugs damage gastroduodenal mucosa through the inhibition of the cyclooxygenase pathway.

INTRODUCTION

Peptic ulcer disease (PUD) is the result of defects in the gastroduodenal mucosa mediated by an imbalance of mucosal protective and mucosal damaging mechanisms, thus leading to ulcer formation. Ulcerations are primarily located in the stomach and duodenum but can also be found in the lower esophagus. Ulcerations vary in size and can be superficial but can cause more extensive disease by extending from the muscularis mucosa into the deeper layers of the mucosa. The cause of PUD was previously thought to be caused by increased gastric acid production, dietary factors, and/or stress. However, with the isolation and identification of the bacterium, *H pylori*, as well as the increased consumption of nonsteroidal antiinflammatory drugs (NSAIDs), evidence has shown that these are the main causes of PUD.[1] However, these factors alone are likely not enough on their own to cause ulcer formation. Other risk factors, including smoking, alcohol use, poor dietary habits, low socioeconomic status, presence of anxiety and stress, cocaine use, exogenous steroid use, advanced age, and Zollinger-Ellison syndrome, may also aid in ulcer formation.[2–4] Fortunately, most of the patients diagnosed with uncomplicated PUD can be treated successfully.[5]

Physician Assistant Program, Baylor College of Medicine, One Baylor Plaza, BCM MS 115, Houston, TX 77030, USA
E-mail address: shell@bcm.edu

Physician Assist Clin 6 (2021) 603–611
https://doi.org/10.1016/j.cpha.2021.05.005
2405-7991/21/© 2021 Elsevier Inc. All rights reserved.

Epidemiology

PUD continues to cause significant morbidity and mortality worldwide, with more than half of the world population infected. It is thought to be responsible for high health care costs of greater than $3 billion annually.[6] In the United States, PUD affects 4.6 million people annually.[7,8] The lifetime prevalence of PUD is estimated as high as 10% and is less prevalent in developed countries.[1] PUD is the most common cause of upper gastrointestinal bleeding in the Western word; a systematic review estimated the annual incidence of hemorrhage at approximately 19 to 57 cases per 100,000 individuals.[9] Other sequelae of PUD includes abdominal pain, gastric outlet obstruction, and ulcer perforation. Together these complications result in approximately 150,000 hospitalizations annually in the United States.[2]

Pathophysiology

The causes of most PUD cases are caused by *H pylori* infection and chronic NSAID use. Most often, infection begins early in childhood and persists for several decades. *H pylori* has 2 main mechanisms of transmission, oral-oral and fecal-oral. Oral-oral transmission is the primary mechanism by which this organism is transmitted and is seen predominantly in developed countries. Infection among members of the same family is common and sharing of utensils during meals seems to the primary mode of transmission, specifically from an adult to a child.[10] Fecal-oral transmission occurs by the ingestion of contaminated water that is commonly found in countries that have poor sanitation.[11]

H pylori is a helical (spiral) gram-negative bacterium that colonizes the surface of gastric epithelial cells and elicits a deleterious inflammatory response and subsequent damage to host cells. Several bacterial virulence factors have been identified that play a role in the pathogenesis of PUD. *H pylori* infection can be categorized into 3 pathogenic processes: colonization, immune escape, and disease induction.[12]

Colonization

The environment of the stomach was believed to be sterile and not conducive for bacterial colonization and growth. However, this was disproved when *H pylori* was isolated from patient stomach biopsies.[13] Successful colonization and subsequent infection can occur for decades in its host and is aided by several virulence factors, including its shape, urease expression, flagella, urease, chemotaxis, adherence to the gastric epithelium, and manipulation of the host cell and evasion of the immune system (**Fig. 1**).[14,15]

H pylori, a neutrophile or an organism that thrives at a neutral pH, must deploy virulence factors to survive the harsh acidic environment of the stomach. Its corkscrew shape, similar to how a screw passes through a cork, provides a mechanical advantage for penetrating the viscous layer of the stomach and allows for continuous mobility through the mucous layer of the stomach to reach the gastric epithelium.[16]

H pylori enters the body through the mouth and travels through the digestive system to infect the stomach where it must survive unfavorable conditions, such as a low pH and exposure to pepsin. The bacterium secretes large amounts of urease to counteract these conditions and to allow for its survival. This surface-bound enzyme provides a protective milieu by catalyzing the hydrolysis of urea to form ammonia and bicarbonate, which is then released into the cytoplasm and periplasm of the bacterium. This neutralizes the acidic environment inside and around the organism and decreases the viscosity of mucus, allowing for easier mobility of bacteria.[17,18]

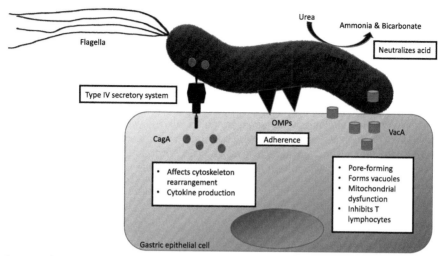

Fig. 1. Pathogenesis of *H pylori*.

The ability of *H pylori* to dynamically modify the host environment and locate to the epithelium is essential to the initial steps of colonization. It must also avoid turnover of the gastric epithelium. To do this, *H pylori* uses a complex motility system and chemosensory-directed motility to efficiently swim through the gastric mucus toward the gastric epithelium. The motility system consists a unipolar bundle of 4 to 8 flagella that rotate in unison to propel the bacterium toward the gastric epithelium and against the rhythmic contractions of the stomach.[19] *H pylori*, in addition to flagella, must sense and integrate signals provided by the gastric epithelium for successful colonization. The ability for the organism to respond to environmental or chemical cues, termed chemotaxis, is orchestrated by core signaling proteins expressed both on the gastric epithelium as well as the bacterium.[20,21]

Under normal physiologic conditions, the epithelial barrier, which consists of gastric epithelial cells, prevents harmful elements in the gastric lumen from having direct access to the mucosa.[22] It is regulated by cell shape, polarity, and intercellular junctions, including tight junctions and cellular interactions with the extracellular matrix. *H pylori*'s attachment to gastric epithelial cells leads to dismantling of the epithelial barrier and is mediated by outer membrane proteins (OMPs).[23] OMPs also help the organism survive the harsh external environment and maintain the integrity of the bacterial cell membrane.[24] OMPs' physical interaction with gastric epithelial cells allows for long-term persistence in the host through gene expression of several bacterial genes.

One of OMPs' essential function is to provide anchorage of a type IV bacterial secretory system to the host cell membrane. The insertion of this system into the host membrane facilitates translocation of bacterial proteins, for example, cytotoxin-gene associated A (CagA), into the host cell.[24,25] Once injected, CagA hijacks host cell machinery and alters several cellular functions leading to dysfunction of the cell.[26] CagA affects cytoskeleton remodeling of the host cell, which leads to aberrant activation of intracellular signaling pathways and elongation of host cells. This may aid in tighter adhesion of the bacterium to gastric epithelial cells and disrupt the integrity of the epithelial barrier.[27,28] CagA is also a potent immunogenic protein and induces the expression of inflammatory cytokines by gastric epithelial cells. The consequence of cytokine production leads to neutrophil migration, infiltration, and heightened inflammation in the stomach, thus contributing to the pathogenesis of disease and ulcer formation.[29–32]

H pylori produces another virulence factor, vacuolating toxin A (VacA), that plays a key role in pathogenesis of disease. VacA, a pore-forming toxin, has diverse biological functions that affect the gastric epithelial cell directly and inhibit T lymphocyte proliferative responses, which will be discussed later. VacA forms pores in the host membrane of the gastric epithelial cell allowing for the transport of vital nutrients, for example, iron and nickel, between intercellular spaces of cells. This process permits *H pylori* access to vital nutrients necessary for its survival within the host.[33] VacA enters the host cell via a receptor-mediated dependent mechanism and induces multiple cellular responses. VacA can form vacuoles inside of the host cell and cause mitochondrial dysfunction, which can lead to apoptosis of the epithelial cell.[34,35] These damaging mechanisms further potentiate a strong inflammatory response that leads to ulcer formation.

Immune Escape

The mammalian immune system consists of 2 tightly coordinated responses, the innate immune response and the adaptive immune response. The innate immune system is the initial response to pathogens and deployed within minutes of detecting a foreign pathogen. It consists of an army of specialized cells, for example, neutrophils, macrophages, and dendritic cells, that are effective at eradicating pathogens. Neutrophils are the first cell type to migrate to the site of infection and drive the inflammatory process, which is necessary to eliminate pathogens. When the innate immune response is unable to combat infection on its own, the adaptive immune response is activated.

The adaptive immune response is tightly regulated and is a highly organized, specific response directed against pathogens. It consists of 2 cell populations, B and T lymphocytes. B lymphocytes produce various antibody subtypes that serve various functions, including neutralizing pathogens, so they no longer have the ability to infect host cells, drive allergic responses, activate the complement system, and activate neutrophils and macrophages to become more efficient at killing pathogens.

T lymphocytes do not produce antibodies and consist of 2 types, CD4+ or T helper lymphocytes and CD8+ T lymphocytes or cytotoxic T lymphocytes (CTLs). T helper cells consist of many different subsets but the 3 most characterized subsets are T helper 1, 2, and 17. T helper 1 lymphocytes are efficient at killing intracellular pathogens, whereas T helper 2 lymphocytes shape B lymphocyte responses, eradicate helminth infections, and are chief contributors to allergic responses and inflammation. T helper 17 cells contribute to inflammation by secreting cytokines, are effective at eradication extracellular pathogens, and are essential in driving efficient mucosal immune responses.

A specialized type of CD4+ T lymphocyte, called regulatory T lymphocytes, police the immune system by suppressing immune responses and limiting the intensity of an immune response. This process is called tolerance and any breakdown in this process leads to the development of autoimmunity.

CTLs are responsible for killing cells infected with pathogens, such as viruses. T helper 1 and T helper 17 lymphocytes have been shown to be important in *H pylori* infection as well as regulatory T lymphocytes. CTLs' role against *H pylori* seems to be minimal.

H pylori has an arsenal of mechanisms to aid in its survival in the host. The bacterium hijacks gastric epithelial cell machinery as well as the immune system. It has also evolved mechanisms to avoid detection by the immune system. The initial defense against *H pylori* infection is the mucus produced by the gastric epithelial cells and the response of the innate immune system present in the lamina propria of the stomach.[36,37] In *H pylori* infection, gastric epithelial cells secrete the cytokine, interleukin-8, which elicits migration of neutrophils to the site of colonization. Neutrophils use a multitude of mechanisms to make them effective at eradicating pathogens.

Recognition of pathogens occurs through toll-like receptors (TLRs), which recognize conserved regions on many different pathogens and are expressed by innate immune cells; this ensures our innate immune system has the capability of recognizing many diverse pathogens. Engagement of these receptors elicits an inflammatory response necessary to eradicate pathogens by recruiting more immune cells to the site of infection. Many organisms, including *H pylori*, have evolved mechanisms to escape TLR recognition.[38] Without engagement of TLRs, the innate immune response will not be able to initiate the appropriate immune response necessary to eradicate infection.

H pylori expresses many different proteins on its cell membrane that help the bacterium escape immune recognition by TLRs persistent in the host. For example, *H pylori* has flagella that rotate in unison to propel the organism toward the gastric epithelium. Flagella are also highly immunogenic; however, *H pylori* can modify its flagella to escape TLR recognition and evade the innate immune response.[39]

H pylori not only has evolved to escape immune recognition by innate immune cells but also has the ability to reshape and avoid detection by the adaptive immune response. *H pylori* infection elicits T helper 1 and 17 responses that are thought to play an essential role in controlling infection; however, *H pylori* uses mechanisms to potentially suppress these responses when these cells migrate to the area of infection.[40–42]

H pylori avoids detection by these T lymphocyte populations by inhibiting T lymphocyte proliferation.[43] VacA seems to play a major role in this inhibitory process by affecting actin rearrangement inside the T lymphocyte, thus inhibiting proliferative responses. VacA forms ion-specific channels, which leads to vacuole formation in T lymphocytes resulting in death. Furthermore, VacA can affect mitochondrial function by causing the release of mitochondrial proapoptotic enzymes in the cytoplasm of T lymphocytes.[44] These mechanisms seem to be the primary mechanism by which *H pylori* mediates suppression of T lymphocyte responses. Without these responses, the bacterium continues to persist in the host and cause chronic infections that lead to peptic ulcer formation and other sequelae.

H pylori not only prevents proliferation of T lymphocytes through several mechanisms previously mentioned but also has the unique ability to skew T lymphocyte responses. Specifically, VacA indirectly drives the differentiation of T helper lymphocytes to regulatory T lymphocytes,[45] and this prevents a robust T lymphocyte response, which allows for *H pylori* to persist in its host.

Bacterial virulence factors and evasion of immune responses permit *H pylori* to cause mucosal damage, thereby leading to an imbalance of mucosal protective and mucosal damaging mechanisms. These processes allow the organism to persist for decades in the host and lead to ulcer formation.

Nonsteroidal Antiinflammatory Drugs

NSAIDs are widely used therapeutics agents because they are effective antipyretics, antiinflammatories, and analgesics. Chronic NSAID use damages the gastroduodenal mucosa through the inhibition of the enzyme cyclooxygenase-1 (COX-1). COX-1 inhibition leads to decreased prostaglandin synthesis inside the cell. Prostaglandins or eicosanoids are a group of lipids derived from arachidonic acid. They regulate homeostatic mechanisms, such as regulate blood flow, inflammation, and platelet aggregation. Reduced mucosal prostaglandin levels result in mucosal damage through decrease mucus and bicarbonate production, which mediate protective roles against the acidity in the stomach.[46] Decreased levels of prostaglandins also result in decreased mucosal blood flow, which is essential in maintaining mucosal integrity. NSAIDs disrupt these homeostatic mechanisms and therefore lead to inflammation, erosions, ulcerations, and bleeding in the stomach.

SUMMARY

PUD continues to be one of the most common diseases worldwide. Various risk factors have been identified for the development of disease but *H pylori* and chronic NSAID use are the most important causes in pathogenesis of disease.

H pylori is one of the most common infections worldwide and has evolved several mechanisms to persist in the host. Increasing antibiotic resistance will pose a problem for future treatment, and therefore, it is key to understand the pathogenesis of disease in order to design effective therapeutics and future vaccines.

CLINICS CARE POINTS

- Peptic ulcer disease is the result of ulcerations in the stomach or duodenum and two primary etiologies include nonsteroidal anti-inflammatory drug use and colonization by the bacterium, Helicobacter pylori.

- Though many patients with uncomplicated peptic ulcer disease may be asymptomatic, those with symptoms most commonly experience classic symptoms, epigastric or retrosternal pain and/or dyspepsia that is relieved or aggravated by consumption of certain liquids, foods, or antacids.

- Non-invasive diagnostic testing for Helicobacter pylori includes urea breath and stool antigen testing; however, patients must discontinue proton pump inhibitors two weeks prior to testing to eliminate the possibility of a false negative test.

- Management of Helicobacter pylori infection takes into account prior antibiotic exposure and first line therapies may include triple or quadruple therapy for 10-14 days.

- Development of resistance to antibiotics is a serious problem and therefore, understanding Helicobacter pylori's virulence factors and the immune response against this organism will lead to the development of novel therapies, e.g., immune modulators, vaccines.

DISCLOSURE

The author has nothing to disclose.

REFERENCES

1. Lanas A, Chan FKL. Peptic ulcer disease. Lancet 2017;390(10094):613–24.
2. Kempenich JW, Sirinek KR. Acid Peptic Disease. Surg Clin North Am 2018;98(5): 933–44.
3. Rosenstock S, Jørgensen T, Bonnevie O, et al. Risk factors for peptic ulcer disease: a population based prospective cohort study comprising 2416 Danish adults. Gut 2003;52(2):186–93.
4. Søreide K, Thorsen K, Harrison EM, et al. Perforated peptic ulcer. Lancet 2015; 386(10000):1288–98.

5. Dunlap JJ, Patterson S. PEPTIC ULCER DISEASE. Gastroenterol Nurs 2019; 42(5):451–4.
6. Peery AF, Crockett SD, Murphy CC, et al. Burden and Cost of Gastrointestinal, Liver, and Pancreatic Diseases in the United States: Update 2018. Gastroenterology 2019;156(1):254–72.e11.
7. Peptic ulcer. OMICS International. Available at: https://www.omicsonline.org/united-states/peptic-ulcer-peer-reviewed-pdf-ppt-articles/. Accessed: October, 2020.
8. Yuan Y, Leontiadis GI. Editorial: ulcer-related vs non-ulcer-nonvariceal upper gastrointestinal bleeding-which has worse outcomes? Aliment Pharmacol Ther 2019;49(6):818–9.
9. Lau JY, Sung J, Hill C, et al. Systematic review of the epidemiology of complicated peptic ulcer disease: incidence, recurrence, risk factors and mortality. Digestion 2011;84(2):102–13.
10. Urita Y, Watanabe T, Kawagoe N, et al. Role of infected grandmothers in transmission of Helicobacter pylori to children in a Japanese rural town. J Paediatr Child Health 2013;49(5):394–8.
11. Goh KL, Chan WK, Shiota S, et al. Epidemiology of Helicobacter pylori infection and public health implications. Helicobacter 2011;16(Suppl 1):1–9.
12. Chang WL, Yeh YC, Sheu BS. The impacts of *H. pylori* virulence factors on the development of gastroduodenal diseases. J Biomed Sci 2018;25(1):68.
13. Warren JR, Marshall B. Unidentified curved bacilli on gastric epithelium in active chronic gastritis. Lancet 1983;1(8336):1273–5.
14. Kao CY, Sheu BS, Wu JJ. Helicobacter pylori infection: An overview of bacterial virulence factors and pathogenesis. Biomed J 2016;39(1):14–23.
15. Sheu BS, Yang HB, Yeh YC, et al. Helicobacter pylori colonization of the human gastric epithelium: a bug's first step is a novel target for us. J Gastroenterol Hepatol 2010;25(1):26–32.
16. Karim QN, Logan RP, Puels J, et al. Measurement of motility of Helicobacter pylori, Campylobacter jejuni, and Escherichia coli by real time computer tracking using the Hobson BacTracker. J Clin Pathol 1998;51(8):623–8.
17. Celli JP, Turner BS, Afdhal NH, et al. Helicobacter pylori moves through mucus by reducing mucin viscoelasticity. Proc Natl Acad Sci U S A 2009;106(34):14321–6.
18. Weeks DL, Eskandari S, Scott DR, et al. A H+-gated urea channel: the link between Helicobacter pylori urease and gastric colonization. Science 2000; 287(5452):482–5.
19. Mobley HLT, Mendz GL, Hazell SL. : Physiology and Genetics. 2001
20. Beier D, Spohn G, Rappuoli R, et al. Identification and characterization of an operon of Helicobacter pylori that is involved in motility and stress adaptation. J Bacteriol 1997;179(15):4676–83.
21. Pittman MS, Goodwin M, Kelly DJ. Chemotaxis in the human gastric pathogen Helicobacter pylori: different roles for CheW and the three CheV paralogues, and evidence for CheV2 phosphorylation. Microbiology (Reading) 2001;147(Pt 9):2493–504.
22. Saadat I, Higashi H, Obuse C, et al. Helicobacter pylori CagA targets PAR1/MARK kinase to disrupt epithelial cell polarity. Nature 2007;447(7142):330–3.
23. Ilver D, Arnqvist A, Ogren J, et al. Helicobacter pylori adhesin binding fucosylated histo-blood group antigens revealed by retagging. Science 1998; 279(5349):373–7.
24. Egan AJF. Bacterial outer membrane constriction. Mol Microbiol 2018;107(6): 676–87.

25. Odenbreit S, Püls J, Sedlmaier B, et al. Translocation of Helicobacter pylori CagA into gastric epithelial cells by type IV secretion. Science 2000;287(5457): 1497–500.
26. Kwok T, Zabler D, Urman S, et al. Helicobacter exploits integrin for type IV secretion and kinase activation. Nature 2007;449(7164):862–6.
27. Yamazaki S, Yamakawa A, Ito Y, et al. The CagA protein of Helicobacter pylori is translocated into epithelial cells and binds to SHP-2 in human gastric mucosa. J Infect Dis 2003;187(2):334–7.
28. Segal ED, Cha J, Lo J, et al. Altered states: involvement of phosphorylated CagA in the induction of host cellular growth changes by Helicobacter pylori. Proc Natl Acad Sci U S A 1999;96(25):14559–64.
29. Yamaoka Y, Kikuchi S, el-Zimaity HM, et al. Importance of Helicobacter pylori oipA in clinical presentation, gastric inflammation, and mucosal interleukin 8 production. Gastroenterology 2002;123(2):414–24.
30. Horridge DN, Begley AA, Kim J, et al. Outer inflammatory protein a (OipA) of Helicobacter pylori is regulated by host cell contact and mediates CagA translocation and interleukin-8 response only in the presence of a functional cag pathogenicity island type IV secretion system. Pathog Dis 2017;11(8):75.
31. Fazeli Z, Alebouyeh M, Rezaei Tavirani M, et al. CagA induced interleukin-8 secretion in gastric epithelial cells. Gastroenterol Hepatol Bed Bench 2016; 9(Suppl1):S42–6.
32. Lee KE, Khoi PN, Xia Y, et al. Helicobacter pylori and interleukin-8 in gastric cancer. World J Gastroenterol 2013;19(45):8192–202.
33. Czajkowsky DM, Iwamoto H, Cover TL, et al. The vacuolating toxin from Helicobacter pylori forms hexameric pores in lipid bilayers at low pH. Proc Natl Acad Sci U S A 1999;96(5):2001–6.
34. Papini E, Zoratti M, Cover TL. In search of the Helicobacter pylori VacA mechanism of action. Toxicon 2001;39(11):1757–67.
35. Cover TL, Krishna US, Israel DA, et al. Induction of gastric epithelial cell apoptosis by Helicobacter pylori vacuolating cytotoxin. Cancer Res 2003;63(5): 951–7.
36. Chmiela M, Karwowska Z, Gonciarz W, et al. Host pathogen interactions in. World J Gastroenterol 2017;23(9):1521–40.
37. Mejías-Luque R, Gerhard M. Immune Evasion Strategies and Persistence of Helicobacter pylori. Curr Top Microbiol Immunol 2017;400:53–71.
38. Stead CM, Beasley A, Cotter RJ, et al. Deciphering the unusual acylation pattern of Helicobacter pylori lipid A. J Bacteriol 2008;190(21):7012–21.
39. Gewirtz AT, Yu Y, Krishna US, et al. Helicobacter pylori flagellin evades toll-like receptor 5-mediated innate immunity. J Infect Dis 2004;189(10):1914–20.
40. Bagheri N, Salimzadeh L, Shirzad H. The role of T helper 1-cell response in Helicobacter pylori-infection. Microb Pathog 2018;123:1–8.
41. Bagheri N, Razavi A, Pourgheysari B, et al. Up-regulated Th17 cell function is associated with increased peptic ulcer disease in Helicobacter pylori-infection. Infect Genet Evol 2018;60:117–25.
42. Sun H, Yuan H, Tan R, et al. Immunodominant antigens that induce Th1 and Th17 responses protect mice against. Oncotarget 2018;9(15):12050–63.
43. Gebert B, Fischer W, Weiss E, et al. Helicobacter pylori vacuolating cytotoxin inhibits T lymphocyte activation. Science 2003;301(5636):1099–102.
44. Abadi ATB. Strategies used by. World J Gastroenterol 2017;23(16):2870–82.

45. Oertli M, Noben M, Engler DB, et al. Helicobacter pylori γ-glutamyl transpepti-dase and vacuolating cytotoxin promote gastric persistence and immune toler-ance. Proc Natl Acad Sci U S A 2013;110(8):3047–52.

46. Bhala N, Emberson J, Merhi A, et al. Vascular and upper gastrointestinal effects of non-steroidal anti-inflammatory drugs: meta-analyses of individual participant data from randomised trials. Lancet 2013;382(9894):769–79.

Refractory Gastroesophageal Reflux Disease: A Closer Look

Jennifer Hastings, MSHS, PA-C

KEYWORDS

- GERD • Refractory GERD • Persistent GERD • GERD management

KEY POINTS

- GERD can manifest in various differing clinical presentations and can lead to significant complications, including esophagitis, strictures, and Barrett esophagus.
- Esophageal carcinoma can present with GERD symptoms.
- Medication compliance in addition to lifestyle and dietary modifications is vital for successful management of GERD.
- Weight loss in patients who are overweight or obese has been shown to significantly reduce GERD symptoms.
- Providers must evaluate for alarm features at each visit and refer patients for endoscopic evaluation appropriately.

INTRODUCTION

Gastroesophageal reflux disease (GERD) is a common pathologic condition that affects approximately 18.1% to 27.8% of the population in North America.[1] GERD has an annual financial burden of approximately $9 to 10 billion dollars in the United States alone.[2]

The American College of Gastroenterology (ACG) practice guidelines for GERD describe GERD as "symptoms or complications resulting from the reflux of gastric contents into the esophagus or beyond, into the oral cavity (including larynx) or lung."[3] As such, GERD can present with esophageal and extraesophageal symptoms. The classic symptoms of GERD include heartburn and reflux. Atypical symptoms of GERD may include nausea, bloating, dyspepsia, dysphagia, epigastric pain, chest pain (noncardiac), and eructation.[1] Patients can also develop extraesophageal manifestations of GERD, including cough, wheezing (asthma), and throat symptoms (hoarseness, pain, or frequent clearing).[1]

Acid suppressants can include antacids, histamine receptor antagonists (H2RA), and proton-pump inhibitors (PPI). PPIs are the strongest of the acid suppressants

Niceville, FL, USA
E-mail address: hastings.jenny@gmail.com

Physician Assist Clin 6 (2021) 613–623
https://doi.org/10.1016/j.cpha.2021.05.006
2405-7991/21/© 2021 Elsevier Inc. All rights reserved.
physicianassistant.theclinics.com

and are used in the management of refractory GERD. Unfortunately, as much as 40% of patients fail treatment with PPI therapy.[3] There is not a universally accepted definition of refractory GERD other than to imply that the patient has persistent GERD symptoms despite treatment with PPI therapy.[3] Sources have defined refractory GERD to include persistent symptoms despite completion of 12 weeks of PPI therapy,[4] whereas others define GERD as refractory when symptoms are still present following 8 weeks of PPI therapy.[1,5]

When evaluating a patient with refractory GERD symptoms, a detailed history must be completed focusing on the presence of alarm symptoms, medication compliance, as well as dietary and lifestyle habits. Patient education is an important part of management in the primary care setting. Recognizing when to refer these patients for endoscopic evaluation is another important aspect of primary care management. Diagnostic evaluation and management of refractory GERD are typically pursued in the specialty setting. There are multiple newer treatment options available for GERD that are briefly reviewed in this article. However, limited long-term data proving safety and efficacy have limited recommendations for widespread use.

IDENTIFYING HIGH-RISK PATIENTS

GERD is often diagnosed with a classic history of heartburn and reflux, and an empiric trial of PPI therapy is recommended. In patients that experience a favorable response, a presumptive diagnosis of GERD is made. This approach is beneficial in low-risk patients, as further diagnostic testing that can be costly and invasive may be avoided. However, this approach does not always correlate with a true presence of GERD.[3] Identifying high-risk patients that should be referred for further evaluation is a key aspect of GERD management in the primary care setting.

GERD is often considered a benign entity. However, GERD can lead to esophageal complications, including esophageal (peptic) strictures, erosive esophagitis, and Barrett esophagus. Individuals with chronic GERD have a 5% to 15% prevalence of underlying Barrett esophagus.[2] Barrett esophagus increases the risk of esophageal adenocarcinoma. Esophageal adenocarcinoma should be included in the differential diagnosis of any patient presenting with GERD symptoms. Men who have history of chronic GERD (at least 5 years) or frequent (at least weekly) GERD symptoms in addition to 2 other risk factors for Barrett esophagus should be referred for baseline upper endoscopy.[6] Additional risk factors for Barrett esophagus include male gender, aged 50 years or older, white race, central obesity, past or present use of tobacco, and family history of Barrett esophagus or esophageal adenocarcinoma in a first-degree relative (Fig. 1).[6]

Initial and all subsequent encounters should include evaluation for alarm features, which, if present, may indicate a more serious underlying diagnosis or complication of GERD. Alarm features in a patient presenting with possible GERD include new symptoms presenting in an older demographic ($\geq$60 years), unintentional weight loss, anorexia, signs of gastrointestinal (GI) bleeding (iron deficiency anemia, hematemesis, melena, hematochezia, hemoccult-positive stool), dysphagia or odynophagia, persistent vomiting, or history of GI malignancy in a first-degree relative (see Fig. 1).[7] Individuals with refractory GERD symptoms should also be referred for further evaluation.[3] The refractory nature in such a scenario can be considered an alarm feature in itself.

Cardiac causes must be considered in patients presenting with chest pain, "heartburn," or other upper GI symptoms. A detailed history paired with assessment of cardiac risk factors should be completed. When cardiac pathologic condition is

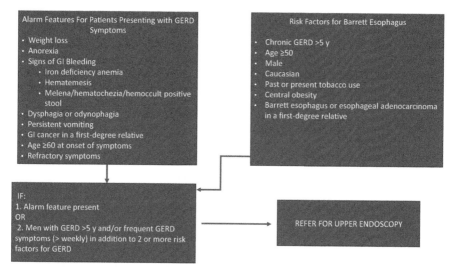

Fig. 1. Identifying high-risk patients requiring endoscopic evaluation. (*Adapted From* Fass, R. Approach to refractory gastroesophageal reflux disease in adults. Talley NH, Grover S, eds. UpToDate.: Waltham, MA; UpToDate. 2020. www.uptodate.com. Accessed, November 15, 2020[7]; and Shaheen, Nicholas J MD, MPH, FACG1; Falk, Gary W MD, MS, FACG2; Iyer, Prasad G MD, MSc, FACG3; Gerson, Lauren B MD, MSc, FACG4 ACG Clinical Guideline: Diagnosis and Management of Barrett's Esophagus, American Journal of Gastroenterology: January 2016 - Volume 111 - Issue 1 - p 30-50 https://doi.org/10.1038/ajg.2015.322.[6])

suspected, a cardiac evaluation should be completed before pursuing endoscopic evaluation.

CLINICS CARE POINTS

- When evaluating a patient with gastroesophageal reflux disease, identify high-risk patients.
- Patients presenting with alarm symptoms suggestive of a potential complication, such as esophageal adenocarcinoma, or risk factors for Barrett esophagus should be referred for upper endoscopy without delay.

REFRACTORY GASTROESOPHAGEAL REFLUX DISEASE: EARLY MANAGEMENT

In patients with refractory GERD, additional diagnostic testing is typically required to establish a more definitive diagnosis, verify effectiveness of treatment, or rule out an alternative diagnosis. However, before the pursuit of further testing or adding therapeutics, it is important to optimize PPI therapy and focus on diet and lifestyle modifications.

Proton-Pump Inhibitors Therapy

Acid-suppressive therapy is the cornerstone of GERD management. PPIs are the most potent of the acid suppressants. PPI therapy has been shown to be superior to H_2RAs in the management of erosive esophagitis as well as nonerosive reflux disease.[3] H_2RAs are often used in individuals with milder disease or as an adjunct to PPI therapy. However, tachyphylaxis can occur with H_2RAs, which can contribute to treatment failure.[5]

Traditionally, PPI therapy is initiated once daily. For patients that are experiencing persistent symptoms despite daily PPI therapy, twice-daily therapy can be recommended or alternatively a trial of a different PPI may be attempted.[3]

Medication compliance and appropriate administration of PPI therapy are important to achieve maximal acid suppression. PPI therapy is best taken 30 to 60 minutes before the first meal of the day, as this is when there is the largest amount of hydrogen-potassium ATP-ase present on the parietal cell leading to higher acid suppression.[8] Patients who require twice-daily dosing should be prompted to take the second dose 30 to 60 minutes before dinner.[8] Of note, PPIs do not provide maximum acid suppression when used on an as-needed basis.

In patients experiencing refractory symptoms, verifying PPI compliance has considerable value, as evidence suggests that PPI misuse is a frequent occurrence. In a study consisting of 100 participants, 54% of patients were determined to be using PPI therapy suboptimally, which included taking PPI therapy greater than 60 minutes before mealtime, as needed, or at nighttime.[9] Of 46% of subjects that were classified as "optimal" dosers, only 17% reported taking PPI therapy within the optimal window of 30 to 60 minutes before mealtime.[9] Patient education regarding appropriate PPI administration should be incorporated into each visit.

Concerns regarding potential side effects of long-term PPI use have been raised, including the increased risk of *Clostridioides difficile* and other enteric infections, osteoporosis or bone fractures, cobalamin and magnesium deficiency, aspiration pneumonia, atrophic gastritis, interstitial nephritis, cardiovascular events in those taking clopidogrel, and dementia.[10] The overall evidence linking most of these potential complications with long-term PPI use is fairly weak.[10] Current recommendations include limiting PPI therapy to the lowest effective dose and the shortest course that symptoms will allow.[1,3,8,10] In certain patients, the benefit of prolonged PPI therapy likely outweighs the risk. Recommendations for long-term PPI use are reserved for individuals with complications secondary to GERD, such as Barrett esophagus, as well as those who are unable to discontinue therapy secondary to an exacerbation of symptoms.[3]

Patient Education: Lifestyle and Diet Modifications

Dietary and lifestyle indiscretion has long been thought to exacerbate GERD. All patients with GERD, regardless of treatment with PPI or other acid-suppressive therapy, should be counseled on diet and lifestyle modifications to reduce symptoms and potentially reduce medication requirements. Making sweeping recommendations to avoid all potential triggers will likely be overwhelming and make it less likely the patient will comply. In addition, the evidence does not support this approach, as a strong connection between dietary modifications and improvement in GERD symptoms has not been established.[11] Focusing on eliminating specific dietary triggers will make it easier for the patient to be successful.

Although cumbersome, in certain patients, a diary documenting eating and sleep habits in addition to symptom timing may aid in the identification of specific triggers in individuals with refractory symptoms. Specific dietary triggers identified should be eliminated from the patient's diet. The most common dietary triggers of GERD include tobacco, alcohol, caffeine, carbonated beverages, chocolate, acidic or citrus foods, fatty foods, spicy foods, and mint.[1] Although the intake of some of these substances has been identified to reduce lower esophageal sphincter (LES) pressure, increase reflux episodes, or increase pH, there is limited evidence that links the actual elimination of these substances with either improvement in symptoms or physiologic factors predisposing to GERD, such as raising esophageal pH or increasing LES pressure.[3,11]

Nighttime eating and drinking can be a significant factor for those experiencing nocturnal symptoms. Recommendations should be made to avoid eating or drinking within 2 to 3 hours of bedtime.[1,3] Elevating the head of the bed and sleeping in the left lateral decubitus position have been shown to decrease the time that the intraeso-phageal pH is less than 4.[11]

Weight Loss

Obesity is an additional well-known risk factor for GERD. Evidence shows that an in-crease in body mass index (BMI) correlates directly with an increase in GERD symp-toms.[12] Weight loss has been shown to be effective in reducing GERD symptoms. In a prospective cohort study, 332 individuals were enrolled in a structured weight loss program over 6 months with 124 subjects identified as having GERD.[13] Over the course of the 6 months, the average weight loss was 13.1 kg, and the average reduc-tion in waist circumference was 10.6 cm. Eighty-one percent reported a reduction in GERD symptoms overall, whereas 65% reported a complete resolution of GERD symptoms.[13] This study also identified a linear relationship between the amount of weight lost and the degree in which GERD symptoms were reduced.[13]

Obesity increases mortality, and the negative health burden of obesity extends far beyond GERD.[14] Weight loss provides a significant reduction of GERD symptoms in addition to numerous other health benefits to include but not limited to lowering cholesterol, lowering blood pressure, improving insulin resistance, lowering blood sugar, reducing cancer risk, improving sleep apnea, reversing hepatic steatosis, improving depression, and reducing stress on weightbearing joints.[14]

The US Preventative Services Task Force recommends that that all patients with a BMI of ≥ 30 be referred for multicomponent behavioral therapy.[15] Behavioral therapy provides a more formalized approach, which often includes counseling, education, support, and tools tailored to individual patient needs to maintain positive lifestyle changes on a long-term basis. Given the significant overall health benefits of weight loss and the reduction of overall mortality paralleled with the proven benefit in pa-tients with GERD, it stands to reason that substantial efforts should be dedicated to successful weight reduction in overweight and obese patients with refractory GERD.

CLINICS CARE POINTS

- Patient education is a key component of gastroesophageal reflux disease management. Patients presenting with gastroesophageal reflux disease or refractory gastroesophageal reflux disease should be counseled on the following:

- Elimination of dietary triggers for gastroesophageal reflux disease.

- Avoidance of eating or drinking within 2 to 3 hours of bedtime.

- Elevating the head of the bed.

- Appropriate administration of proton-pump inhibitors therapy (30–60 minutes before the first meal of the day).

- Given the significant association between weight loss and improvement of gastroesophageal reflux disease symptoms, patients who are overweight or obese should be counseled on weight loss measures.

REFRACTORY GASTROESOPHAGEAL REFLUX DISEASE: EVALUATION
Upper Endoscopy

Patients with alarm features or risk factors for Barrett esophagus, and individuals experiencing refractory GERD symptoms warrant investigation. An upper endoscopy should be completed to evaluate response to treatment, identify complications, and assess for evidence of an alternative diagnosis.

Endoscopic findings of erosive esophagitis (known as erosive reflux disease), peptic stricture, or Barrett esophagus confirm a diagnosis of GERD.[3] An upper endoscopy does not always confirm a diagnosis of GERD. Most often, patients with GERD have normal-appearing esophageal mucosa without evidence of erosions, nonerosive reflux disease, in which case the diagnosis may remain in question.[3] An esophageal biopsy completed at the time of endoscopy can rule out diagnoses such as eosino-philic esophagitis.

Esophageal pH and Impedance-pH Testing

Further investigation and confirmation of a GERD diagnosis can be completed with pH testing via wireless pH capsule, or via an intranasal pH probe or dual impedance-pH monitoring.[7] Dual impedance-pH monitoring collects additional useful information. This study is beneficial, as it captures both the intraesophageal pH (the presence of acid) in addition to esophageal impedance (reflux episodes). The investigator can determine if the patient has a correlation between acid or nonacid reflux episodes and symptoms.

Studies using esophageal impedance-pH testing have demonstrated that very few patients taking twice-daily PPI therapy continue to experience symptoms secondary to breakthrough acid reflux, confirming adequate acid suppression for most patients. However, patients can experience symptoms secondary to nonacid reflux, as mechanisms predisposing the individual to regurgitation are likely still present (hiatal hernia, obesity, dysmotility, or abnormal LES relaxation).[7] In a study of 168 patients who were taking at least twice-daily PPI therapy for a month or more, only 11% were found to have symptoms that correlated with breakthrough acid exposure on dual esophageal impedance-pH monitoring.[16] In this same study, 37% were determined to have a positive correlation between reported symptoms and nonacid reflux episodes.[16]

Esophageal Manometry

Patients experiencing dysphagia or atypical chest pain without significant findings on endoscopy should be considered for esophageal manometry to rule out an esophageal motility disorder, such as achalasia or diffuse esophageal spasm. In addition, if an antireflux procedure is being considered, an esophageal manometry is required before surgery.

ALTERNATIVE DIAGNOSIS: A REVIEW

Following specialty evaluation, the differential diagnosis for refractory GERD should be narrowed with the exclusion of diagnoses, such as esophageal malignancy and eosinophilic esophagitis, with completion of an upper endoscopy. In patients with chest pain and/or dysphagia, esophageal manometry will evaluate for any motility disorders.

The most common causes of refractory heartburn are the functional disorders, reflux hypersensitivity and functional heartburn, which present with normal-appearing esophageal mucosa.[1,17] These diagnoses can be made based on results of esophageal impedance-pH testing. Reflux hypersensitivity is suspected when the patient meets the criteria for normal pH testing but has a positive correlation between heartburn or substernal symptoms and normal physiologic acid or weak acid reflux episodes.[7,17] Specifically, patients with reflux hypersensitivity are sensitive to the presence of small amounts of acid or weak acid in the esophagus that are otherwise considered to be nonpathologic.

Functional heartburn is considered when the patient is experiencing heartburn or retrosternal discomfort with normal pH testing and no symptom correlation with reflux episodes.[7] Individuals with functional esophageal disorders, such as reflux hypersensitivity and functional heartburn, tend to have a higher incidence of other functional disorders and psychological disorders, such as anxiety and depression.[17] Pain modulators, such as selective serotonin reuptake inhibitors, tricyclic antidepressants, serotonin norepinephrine reuptake inhibitors, and trazodone, may provide benefit for patients with either esophageal hypersensitivity or functional heartburn.[1,7,17]

MEDICAL MANAGEMENT OF REFRACTORY GASTROESOPHAGEAL REFLUX DISEASE

By definition, individuals with refractory GERD have continued symptoms despite a trial of twice-daily PPI therapy. As discussed, few patients on twice-daily PPI therapy have actual breakthrough acid reflux based on pH testing. For individuals with suspected breakthrough nighttime symptoms, an H_2RA can be added at bedtime. Of note, given the potential for tachyphylaxis, an alternative may include the addition of a nighttime H_2RA as needed with dietary indiscretion or when experiencing increased symptoms.[3]

Baclofen, a $GABA_B$ receptor agonist, is a reflux inhibitor that is thought to limit relaxations of the LES and reduce reflux (both acid and nonacid reflux).[18] Baclofen is not Food and Drug Administration approved for the treatment of GERD and is typically only considered in the specialty setting for patients that continue to have severe refractory reflux (either acid or nonacid) identified on evaluation that has persisted despite maximum acid suppression.[1] Baclofen does require close monitoring, as it crosses the blood-brain barrier and increases the risk of symptoms such as drowsiness and dizziness.

Metoclopramide is a prokinetic agent effective in the management of gastroparesis and is occasionally considered for severe refractory GERD (most likely in the specialty setting). Metoclopramide has some favorable effects that may benefit GERD, including the enhancement of gastric emptying; however, the use of metoclopramide is significantly limited because of the risk of worrisome neurologic side effects, such as tardive dyskinesia.[3]

ANTIREFLUX PROCEDURES

Antireflux procedures for the management of GERD are typically reserved for those with severe refractory GERD despite PPI therapy. However, given recent concerns regarding the safety of prolonged PPI use, some patients may wish to circumvent the need for PPI therapy indefinitely.

There is always concern for surgical complications and postoperative symptoms with invasive procedures. The most significant and frequent postoperative symptoms reported following antireflux procedures include dysphagia, the inability to vomit or belch, gas, and bloat. Significant measures of procedure success are reduction in GERD symptoms, the absence of procedure-related symptoms or complications, and the ability to remain off PPI therapy.

Antireflux procedures for the management of GERD have expanded beyond the gold-standard fundoplication over recent years to include magnetic sphincter augmentation devices (MSAD, LINX, Shoreview, Minnesota), endoscopic radiofrequency antireflux procedure (Stretta, RESTECH, Houston, Texas), and transoral incisionless fundoplication (EsophyX). These newer procedures are typically performed in specialty settings, are not universally available, and have limited insurance coverage. Although these newer treatment modalities have shown some promise in the management of GERD, there is concern regarding long-term efficacy and safety. The ACG practice guidelines for GERD do not recommend alternative endoscopic or surgical modalities in place of traditional therapies, such as fundoplication and PPI therapy.[3]

Nissen Fundoplication

Certain individuals with GERD are more favorable surgical candidates. Patients with typical GERD symptoms that are responsive to PPI therapy in addition to individuals that have abnormalities on pH testing correlating with their symptoms have been identified as the cohort most likely to benefit from fundoplication.[3] Alternatively, individuals with atypical/extraesophageal symptoms and those that have not experienced benefit from PPI therapy are less likely to benefit from fundoplication.[3]

Laparoscopic Nissen fundoplication remains the gold-standard antireflux procedure.[19] Fundoplication is the oldest antireflux procedure, which provides the ability to investigate long-term outcomes in comparison to some of the newer treatment modalities. One long-term randomized controlled prospective study of 86 patients compared laparoscopic versus open fundoplication outcomes over 15 years. At the 15-year follow-up, 76.7% of all patients were asymptomatic or only mildly symptomatic, whereas 10.5% reported difficult heartburn or regurgitation symptoms.[19] In addition, 67.5% of patients overall denied having any dysphagia, whereas 3.5% reported "severe or difficult" dysphagia with improvement of dysphagia prevalence over time.[19] Overall, 43% of patients reported disturbing bloating or flatulence. Finally, PPI use was reported to increase over time with 46.5% of all patients returning to PPI use by the 15-year follow-up. There was no significant statistical difference in symptomatic outcome or postoperative symptoms between the open and laparoscopic treatment groups.[20]

Based on the available data, most patients experience benefit from fundoplication. However, the potential for surgical complications, postoperative symptoms, and the moderate likelihood of requiring PPI therapy postprocedure often leads to recommendations for fundoplication only in patients who have the most severe refractory symptoms.

Magnetic Sphincter Augmentation Device

The MSAD (LINX) was approved in 2012 and is a device that is typically placed laparoscopically, using a ring of magnetic beads around the LES to raise the LES pressure and reduce reflux episodes. As the MSAD is a newer modality, long-term treatment and safety outcomes are minimal. There are studies showing a favorable outcome comparable to fundoplication for most patients.[20–22] Available studies of MSAD show approximately 1.1% to 6.7% requiring removal of the device secondary to persistent GERD symptoms or complications, such as esophageal erosion or dysphagia.[23]

Stretta

The Stretta is an endoscopic procedure that was introduced in 2000 for the management of refractory GERD. This procedure delivers radiofrequency energy to the distal esophagus, causing modification to the LES, resulting in increased resting LES pressure and subsequent decreased reflux.[24]

The Stretta procedure has shown promise as an alternative to antireflux surgery with studies demonstrating improvement in parameters, such as reduction in overall PPI use and improved Gastroesophageal Reflux Disease-Health Related Quality of Life score.[24,25] In a meta-analysis of 26 studies, including a total of 2468 Stretta procedures, an overall complication rate of 0.93% was identified.[25] The most common adverse events reported were esophageal erosions and esophageal lacerations. Although there have been some favorable outcomes for the Stretta procedure, there is a call for more quality randomized control trials demonstrating safety and efficacy of Stretta before recommending as alternative over other proven GERD therapies.[3,26]

Transoral Incisionless Fundoplication

Transoral incisionless fundoplication is an additional newer antireflux procedure that creates a partial fundoplication endoscopically.[27] This procedure does show some favorable short-term outcomes in favor of GERD management. However, there is concern, as these effects have been shown to reduce over time.[27] In addition, there are limited prolonged data given the novelty of the procedure leaving long-term efficacy in question. Last, there is risk of serious complications, such as esophageal perforation. Laparoscopic fundoplication is still the recommended first-line antireflux procedure.[27]

CLINICS CARE POINTS

- Twice-daily proton-pump inhibitors therapy typically provides adequate acid suppression for most patients when taken accurately. Patients experiencing refractory gastroesophageal reflux disease (symptoms despite proton-pump inhibitors therapy) should be referred for endoscopic evaluation.

- Specialty evaluation in patients with refractory gastroesophageal reflux disease will assist in identifying alterative diagnosis. Two of the most common causes of refractory heartburn symptoms are functional heartburn and hypersensitive esophagus, which may benefit from pain modulation therapy, as they are functional disorders.

- Antireflux procedures are typically reserved for patients with severe symptoms refractory to proton-pump inhibitors therapy. Nissen fundoplication is considered the gold-standard antireflux procedure.

SUMMARY

Refractory GERD is a common entity with up to 40% of patients experiencing persistent symptoms despite PPI therapy. Recognizing patients with alarm symptoms or who are at risk of complications and in need of endoscopic evaluation is an important component of early management. Focusing on appropriate use of acid suppressive therapy, focusing on weight loss management, and review of lifestyle and diet modifications remain the cornerstone of managing GERD patients.

Patients who experience ongoing GERD symptoms despite compliance with PPI therapy should be referred for further evaluation, including upper endoscopy. Esophageal impedance-pH testing aids in the diagnosis of GERD and the correlation of symptoms with the presence of acid or nonacid reflux.

For patients with severe refractory GERD, antireflux procedures are an option. Laparoscopic Nissen fundoplication remains the gold-standard antireflux procedure. Newer endoscopic and surgical modalities have become available over the past couple of decades, showing promise for GERD management; however, they are not currently recommended over fundoplication or acid suppressive therapy because of limited long-term data proving safety and efficacy.

DISCLOSURE

The author has no commercial or financial conflicts of interest.

REFERENCES

1. Sandhu DS, Fass R. Current trends in the management of gastroesophageal reflux disease. Gut Liver 2018;12(1):7–16.
2. Gyawali CP, Kahrilas PJ, Savarino E, et al. Modern diagnosis of GERD: the Lyon consensus. Gut 2018;67(7):1351–62.
3. Katz PO, Gerson LB, Vela MF. Guidelines for the diagnosis and management of gastroesophageal reflux disease. Am J Gastroenterol 2013;108(3):308–28.
4. Mermelstein J, Chait Mermelstein A, Chait MM. Proton pump inhibitor-refractory gastroesophageal reflux disease: challenges and solutions. Clin Exp Gastroenterol 2018;11:119–34.
5. Young A, Kumar MA, Thota PN. GERD: a practical approach. Cleve Clin J Med 2020;87(4):223–30.
6. Shaheen NJ, Falk GW, Iyer PG, et al. ACG clinical guideline: diagnosis and management of Barrett's esophagus. Am J Gastroenterol 2016;111(1):30–50.
7. Fass R. Approach to refractory gastroesophageal reflux disease in adults. In: Talley NH, Grover S, editors. UpToDate. Waltham (MA): UpToDate; 2020. Available at: www.uptodate.com. Accessed November 15, 2020.
8. Schnoll-Sussman F, Niec R, Katz P. Proton pump inhibitors. Gastrointest Endosc Clin N Am 2020;30(2):239–51.
9. Gunaratnam NT, Jessup TP, Inadomi J, et al. Sub-optimal proton pump inhibitor dosing is prevalent in patients with poorly controlled gastro-oesophageal reflux disease. Aliment Pharmacol Ther 2006;23(10):1473–7.
10. Freedberg DE, Kim LS, Yang Y-X. The risks and benefits of long-term use of proton pump inhibitors: expert review and best practice advice from the American Gastroenterological Association. Gastroenterology 2017;152(4):706–15.
11. Kaltenbach T, Crockett S, Gerson LB. Are lifestyle measures effective in patients with gastroesophageal reflux disease? An evidence-based approach. Arch Intern Med 2006;166(9):965–71.
12. Jacobson BC, Somers SC, Fuchs CS, et al. Body-mass index and symptoms of gastroesophageal reflux in women. N Engl J Med 2006;354(22):2340–8.
13. Singh M, Lee J, Gupta N, et al. Weight loss can lead to resolution of gastroesophageal reflux disease symptoms: a prospective intervention trial. Obesity 2013; 21(2):284–90.
14. Soleymani T, Daniel S, Garvey W. Weight maintenance: challenges, tools and strategies for primary care physicians. Obes Rev 2015;17(1):81–93.
15. United States Preventive Service Task Force. Weight loss to prevent obesity-related morbidity and mortality in adults: behavioral interventions. 2018. Available at: https://www.uspreventiveservicestaskforce.org/uspstf/recommendation/obesity-in-adults-interventions. Accessed: December 5, 2020.
16. Mainie I, Tutuian R, Shay S, et al. Acid and non-acid reflux in patients with persistent symptoms despite acid suppressive therapy: a multicentre study using combined ambulatory impedance-pH monitoring. Gut 2006;55(10):1398–402.
17. Yamasaki T, Fass R. Reflux hypersensitivity: a new functional esophageal disorder. J Neurogastroenterol Motil 2017;23(4):495–503.
18. Cossentino MJ, Mann K, Armbruster SP, et al. Randomised clinical trial: the effect of baclofen in patients with gastro-oesophageal reflux–a randomised prospective study. Aliment Pharmacol Ther 2012;35(9):1036–44.

19. Salminen P, Hurme S, Ovaska J. Fifteen-year outcome of laparoscopic and open Nissen fundoplication: a randomized clinical trial. Ann Thorac Surg 2012;93(1): 228–33.
20. Riegler M, Schoppman SF, Bonavina L, et al. Magnetic sphincter augmentation and fundoplication for GERD in clinical practice: one-year results of a multicenter, prospective observational study. Surg Endosc 2015;29:1123–9.
21. Louie BE, Smith CD, Smith CC, et al. Objective evidence of reflux control after magnetic sphincter augmentation: one year results from a post approval study. Ann Surg 2019;270(2):302–8.
22. Bonavina L, Horbach T, Schoppmann SF, et al. Three-year clinical experience with magnetic sphincter augmentation and laparoscopic fundoplication. Surg Endosc 2020. https://doi.org/10.1007/s00464-020-07792-1.
23. Tatum JM, Alicuben E, Bildzukewicz N, et al. Removing the magnetic sphincter augmentation device: operative management and outcomes. Surg Endosc 2019;33:2663–9.
24. Noar M, Squires P, Noar E, et al. Long-term maintenance effect of radiofrequency energy delivery for refractory GERD: a decade later. Surg Endosc 2014;28(8): 2323–33.
25. Fass R, Cahn F, Scotti DJ, et al. Systematic review and meta-analysis of controlled and prospective cohort efficacy studies of endoscopic radiofrequency for treatment of gastroesophageal reflux disease. Surg Endosc 2017;31(12): 4865–82.
26. Lipka S, Kumar A, Richter JE. No evidence for efficacy of radiofrequency ablation for treatment of gastroesophageal reflux disease: a systematic review and meta-analysis. Clin Gastroenterol Hepatol 2015;13(6):1058–67.e1.
27. Richter JE, Kumar A, Lipka S, et al. Efficacy of laparoscopic Nissen fundoplication vs transoral incisionless fundoplication or proton pump inhibitors in patients with gastroesophageal reflux disease: a systematic review and network meta-analysis. Gastroenterology 2018;154(5):1298–308.e7.

Updated Screening Strategies for Colorectal Cancer

Tina M. Butler, DMSc, MPAS, PA-C*

KEYWORDS

- Colorectal cancer screening • Colorectal cancer • FIT testing • Colonoscopy

KEY POINTS

- Colorectal cancer is the third leading cause of cancer-related death in men and women.
- Colorectal cancer screening is cost-effective and cost saving.
- Viable screening options include annual or biennial stool-based tests, flexible sigmoidoscopy every 5 to 10 years, and colonoscopy every 10 years.
- Increasing awareness, shared decision-making, and helping patients overcome barriers to screening can improve colorectal cancer screening rates and save lives.

INTRODUCTION

According to the American Cancer Society, colorectal cancer (CRC) is the third most common cancer diagnosed in both men and women, is the third leading cause of cancer-related deaths in men and women, and is the second most common cause of cancer death when men and women are combined.[1] In 2017, 141,425 new cases of CRC were reported and 52,547 people died.[2] CRS affects men and women of all racial and ethnic groups, and it is most commonly diagnosed in individuals 50 years of age or older.[3] The American Cancer Society estimates in 2020, there will be 104,610 new cases for colon cancer, 43,340 new cases for rectal cancer, and 53,200 deaths.[1] In 2017, the total direct medical costs for cancer including inpatient and outpatient care was $105.5 billion.[4]

Adequate screening is important to reduce CRC incidence and decrease mortality. In the United States, multiple organizations and task forces have created screening guidelines to aid medical providers and increase the number of individuals who are being screened. The goal from the Healthy People 2020 initiative was to have 70.5% of adults aged 50 to 75 years undergo screening for CRC.[5] In 2018, 68.8% of adults aged

Hardin-Simmons University Physician Assistant Program, 2200 Hickory Street, HSU Box 16236, Abilene, TX 79698, USA
* Corresponding author.
E-mail address: tina.butler@hsutx.edu

Physician Assist Clin 6 (2021) 625–635
https://doi.org/10.1016/j.cpha.2021.05.007
2405-7991/21/© 2021 Elsevier Inc. All rights reserved.

Table 1	
Healthy People 2020 goal for CRC screening compared with actual screening rates	
Colorectal Cancer (CRC) Screening Rates for Average-Risk[a] Adults Aged 50–75 y	
Healthy People 2020 Goal	Current CRC Screening Rates
70.5%	Overall = 60%–68.8%
	Latinos = 42%–47.5%
	African Americans = 55.5%

[a] Average risk is defined as an asymptomatic individual without a personal history of CRC, polyps, inflammatory bowel disease, suspected hereditary CRC syndrome, or radiation to the abdomen or pelvis and no family history of CRC.

50 to 75 years were up to date with CRC screening, and 21.7 million adults in the same age range have never been screened[3] (**Table 1**). The focus of this publication is to review the recommendations for CRC screening in average-risk adults while considering the efficacy of the screening modality, cost-effectiveness of screening, barriers and disparities to screening, and strategies to improve screening rates. Individuals are considered average-risk if they do not have a personal history of CRC or polyps, a family history of CRC, a personal history of inflammatory bowel disease, a confirmed or suspected hereditary CRC syndrome, or a personal history of radiation to the abdomen or pelvis to treat a previous cancer.[6]

Colorectal Cancer Screening Guidelines

In the United States, CRC screening guidelines for average-risk adults have been established by the US Preventive Services Task Force (USPSTF), the American College of Gastroenterology (ACG), the American College of Physicians (ACP), and the United States Multi-Society Task Force of Colorectal Cancer Guidelines (MSTF). Unfortunately, these organizations and task forces do not agree on when to start screening, how often screening should occur, which method should be used to screen, and when to stop screening. Having multiple guidelines to reference can be confusing for health care providers and patients.

The USPSTF recommends screening average-risk adults beginning at the age of 50 years and continuing until age 75 years.[7] Screening in adults 76 to 85 years of age should be individualized considering the patient's overall health and history of prior screening.[7] The USPSTF does not endorse a particular screening test to use but instead offers information on all screening options including information on sensitivity and specificity. Recommended screening intervals include annual high-sensitivity guaiac-based fecal occult blood test (gFOBT), annual fecal immunochemical test (FIT), stool FIT-DNA (FIT-DNA) test every 1 to 3 years, flexible sigmoidoscopy (FS) every 5 years, colonoscopy every 10 years, computed tomography (CT) colonography every 5 years, or a combination of FS every 10 years with annual FIT[8] (**Table 2**).

CRC screening for average-risk adults from the ACG clarifies prevention tests from detection tests.[8] Prevention tests include FS, colonoscopy, and CT colonography, and they allow providers to identify precancerous lesions.[8] Detection tests include all fecal tests, which as a whole have lower sensitivity for adenomatous polyp detection when compared with prevention tests.[8] The ACG initially recommends screening with colonoscopy in average-risk adults starting at age 50 years and in African Americans starting at age 45 years.[8] Should colonoscopy not be available or the patient refuses colonoscopy, then the ACG recommends another prevention test such as FS every 5 to 10 years or CT colonography every 5 years.[8] If the patient refuses any of

Table 2
Overview of the colorectal cancer screening recommendations from the US Preventive Services Task Force

USPSTF Colorectal Cancer Screening Guidelines					
Age	Start age 50 y; stop age 75 y				
	76–85 y should be individualized based on risk and previous screening				
Recommended Screening Modalities[a]					
Annual gFOBT or	Annual FIT or	FIT-DNA every 1–3 y or	FS every 5 y or	Colonoscopy every 10 y or	CT colonography every 5 y

[a] No screening modality recommended over another.

the prevention tests, then the recommended detection-based tests are either annual FIT or FIT-DNA every 3 years[8] (**Table 3**).

The ACP recommends screening average-risk adults beginning at age 50 years through age 75 years using one of the following 4 tests: high-sensitivity FOBT or FIT annually, FS every 5 years, colonoscopy every 10 years, or a combination of high-sensitivity FOBT or FIT every 3 years and FS every 5 years.[8] Similar to the USPSTF, the ACP does not recommend one test over any of the others. For individuals older than 75 years who have a life expectancy less than 10 years, CRC screening is not recommended[8] (**Table 4**).

The United States Multi-Society Task Force of Colorectal Cancer Guidelines represents the combined work from the ACG, the American Gastroenterological Association, and the American Society for Gastrointestinal Endoscopy. MSTF makes a distinction between screening, diagnostic examinations, and surveillance. Surveillance uses colonoscopy in set intervals in patients with known CRC or precancerous lesions, which is not the focus of this paper.[9] Diagnostic examinations are used when patients either have symptoms or a positive screening test, with colonoscopy being the diagnostic examination of choice.[9] Screening used in the United States is through the opportunistic approach where providers use several broad strategies to offer screening either through multiple options (test A vs test B) or in a sequential approach (patient refuses test A, offer test B).[9] The MSTF recommends screening begin at age 50 years and end at age 75 years for average-risk individuals using multiple or sequential screening options.[9] Initiation of CRC screening for African Americans is recommended to start at age 45 years.[9] The MSTF recommendations are organized in a 3-tier manner with considerations based on performance, costs, and practical considerations. Tier 1 recommends CRC screening with colonoscopy every 10 years along with annual FIT testing.[9] In patients who refuse Tier 1 options, then Tier 2 options include CT colonography every 5 years, or FIT-DNA every 3 years, or FS every 5 to 10 years.[9] Tier 3 recommendation is capsule colonoscopy every 5 years, but only when the patient declines options from Tier 1 or Tier 2.[9] **Table 5** shows recommendations from MSTF, whereas **Table 6** shows the screening recommendations from all 4 organizations.

Colorectal Cancer Screening Modalities

As noted earlier, there are multiple CRC screening modalities that may be used. In addition to referencing evidence-based guidelines, knowledge of the recommended screening method is important when discussing screening options with patients. Providers should be well versed in explaining the risk versus benefits of each screening modality, along with a clear understanding of the sensitivity and specificity of the

Table 3
Overview of the colorectal cancer screening recommendations from the American College of Gastroenterology

American College of Gastroenterology Colorectal Cancer Screening Guidelines for Average-Risk[a] Adults		
Age	Begin at age 50 y, except in African Americans begin at age 45 y	
Recommended Screening Modalities		
Detection Tests[b]	Annual FIT **or** FIT-DNA every 3 y	
Prevention Tests	Colonoscopy[c] every 10 y **or**	FS every 5–10 y **or**	CT colonography every 5 y

[a] Average-risk is defined as an asymptomatic individual without a personal history of CRC, polyps, inflammatory bowel disease, suspected hereditary CRC syndrome, or radiation to the abdomen or pelvis and no family history of CRC.
[b] Detection tests are recommended as second-line screening modality after all prevention tests have been offered.
[c] Recommended initial screening modality.

test. CRC screening modalities can be categorized as stool-based tests, direct visualization tests, and serology tests.

The intent of stool-based tests is to discover occult blood in the stool in asymptomatic individuals. Stool-based tests include gFOBT, FIT, and FIT-DNA. Multiple randomized clinical trials (RCTs) demonstrate annual or biennial CRC screening with gFOBT reduces CRC deaths,[10] and it is both cost-effective and cost saving.[11] Patients are encouraged to avoid red meats and high-peroxidase fruit and vegetables (turnips, horseradish, and melons) to improve specificity.[12] FITs identify intact human hemoglobin in stool and have better sensitivity over gFOBT for detecting CRC.[10] There is better patient adherence with FIT when compared with gFOBT because there are no dietary restrictions.[8] FIT-DNA is an emerging screening strategy that combines traditional FIT with testing for altered DNA biomarkers.[7] It is commercially known as Cologuard, and it has statistically significant increased sensitivity when compared with FIT alone.[7] An entire stool sample must be collected for analysis, not just a small sample placed on a card (gFOBT or FIT). To date, no longitudinal follow-up data exist for a positive FIT-DNA test with a subsequent negative colonoscopy screen.[7]

Results of multiple randomized control trials showed biennial screening with gFOBT "resulted in reduction in CRC-specific mortality after two to nine rounds of screening (relative risk [RR] 0.91; 95% CI 0.84 to 0.98) at 19.5 years" and annual screening resulted in greater reductions after 11 rounds than biennial screening at 30 years did.[10] Harms associated with stool-based testing is a direct result of additional invasive testing in response to a positive result. The specificity of FIT-DNA is lower than that of FIT alone, thereby increasing the risk for false-positive results.[7] Stool tests that maximize sensitivity have lower specificity, and additional studies are needed to better appreciate the tradeoff of higher false-positive findings.[10]

Direct visualization tests include FS, colonoscopy, and CT colonography. Flexible sigmoidoscopy uses a sigmoidoscope to evaluate the rectum and distal third of the colon. Randomized control trials show a reduction in the incidence and/or mortality of distal and rectosigmoid cancers with FS use[9] and lower CRC-specific mortality compared with no screening at 11 to 12 years follow-up.[10] The reduced mortality benefit with FS, however, is reduced to the distal colon and rectum.[10] Studies also demonstrate combined use of FS (every 5 to 10 years) with FIT (annually) has lower CRC mortality than FS only (hazard ratio 0.62, 95% confidence interval [CI] 0.42–0.90).[10] Despite the

Table 4 Overview of the colorectal cancer screening recommendations from the American College of Physicians			
American College of Physicians Colorectal Cancer Screening Guidelines for Average-Risk[a] Adults			
Age	Start age 50 y; stop age 75 y		
	Age >75 y with a life expectancy <10 y screening not recommended		
Recommended Screening Modalities[b]			
Annual gFOBT or FIT **or**	FS every 5 y **or**	Colonoscopy every 10 y **or**	gFOBT or FIT every 3 y and FS every 5 y

[a] Average-risk is defined as an asymptomatic individual without a personal history of CRC, polyps, inflammatory bowel disease, suspected hereditary CRC syndrome, or radiation to the abdomen or pelvis and no family history of CRC.
[b] No screening modality recommended over another.

documented risk reduction with FS screening, use in the United States has steadily declined in popularity.[9]

Colonoscopy allows for complete examination of the colon, has documented high sensitivity for identification of precancerous and cancerous lesions, and long intervals (10 years) between testing in patients with normal examinations.[9] Disadvantages for colonoscopy include the need for a thorough bowel prep, increased risk for bowel perforation when compared with other screening tests, and greater risk for postprocedural bleeding.[9] According to a systematic review and meta-analysis performed by Fitzpatriz-Lewis and colleagues, no RCTs showed evidence for the benefits of CRC screening by colonoscopy, but several modeling studies predicted an 81% decrease in CRC incidence and an 83% reduction in CRC mortality for average-risk 50-year-olds.[13] Comparatively, stool-based tests showed a 44% to 65% reduction in CRC mortality with gFOBT and 55% to 74% reduction in CRC mortality with FIT, thereby supporting colonoscopy every 10 years.[13]

CT colonography uses low-dose radiation via CT scanning to obtain a minimally invasive view of the colon,[14] but no evidence has found the effectiveness of it as an initial screen.[13] Because of the nature of the examination, CT colonography commonly results in the detection of extracolonic findings in 40% to 70% of screens, with 5% to 37% resulting in additional diagnostic follow-up.[7] Additional diagnostic follow-up may include patients requiring a colonoscopy, an invasive test that requires an additional bowel prep regimen.

The only Food and Drug Administration–approved serology test is designed to detect methylated SEPT9 DNA where SEPT9 gene methylation is associated with the pathogenesis of CRC.[15] However, the SEPT9 DNA test was shown to have low sensitivity for detecting CRC.[7]

Decision Aids

Deciding which CRC screening modality to use is multifactorial. Providers need to consider the cost-effectiveness of the screening test as well as barriers to screening. In addition, patient-related factors due to preference, ethnicity, and special circumstances involved with different vulnerable populations also requires consideration.

Care for individuals with CRC costs the US health care system approximately $14 billion annually.[16] When compared with no screening, colonoscopy every 10 years, FS every 5 years, and yearly gFOBT or FIT examinations were all found to be cost-effective and cost saving for average-risk adults beginning at age 50 years.[17] The American Cancer Society recommends beginning CRC screening at the age of 45

Table 5		
Overview of the colorectal cancer screening recommendations from the US Multi-Society Task Force of Colorectal Cancer Guidelines		
US Multi-Society Task Force of Colorectal Cancer Guidelines for Average-Risk[a] Adults		
Age	50–75 y using multiple or sequential screening options, except African Americans being at age 45 y	
Tier 1	Colonoscopy every 10 y with annual FIT	
Tier 2	CT colonography every 5 y **or** FIT-DNA every 3 y **or** FS every 5–10 y	
Tier 3	Capsule colonoscopy every 5 y	

[a] Average risk is defined as an asymptomatic individual without a personal history of CRC, polyps, inflammatory bowel disease, suspected hereditary CRC syndrome, or radiation to the abdomen or pelvis and no family history of CRC.

years instead of 50 years because deaths from CRC have increased 1% per year from 2008 to 2017.[1] Ladabaum and colleagues compared screening strategies with cost savings using the validated Markov model. Their research found that starting CRC screening at age 45 years is likely to be cost-effective; however, a greater benefit could be achieved by increasing screening rates for unscreened and higher-risk individuals.[18] Specifically, improving screening rates to 80% in patients 50 to 75 years of age would prevent 3 times as many CRC deaths at one-third of the cost.[18]

Patient preferences play a significant role when choosing a CRC screening modality. Test accuracy is ranked by both African Americans and Latinos as an important attribute regardless of the preferred test.[16] African Americans are concerned about discomfort, potential complications, and are more likely to be embarrassed by stool-based DNA testing when compared with whites.[16] Korean Americans have the strongest desire to learn from education sessions whereas Latinos prefer information directly from providers, health brochures, media, and those who speak the same language.[16] Shared decision-making is important for both African Americans and Latinos when compared with whites.[16] In rural populations, screening costs and follow-up costs are more important than travel time or the recommended test modality.[16] Of note, studies have not specifically addressed patients with disabilities or members of the LGBTQIA community.[16]

When assessing the cost-effectiveness of a screening modality, patient adherence also needs to be addressed. Although colonoscopy is considered the gold standard for CRC screening due to its high sensitivity, specificity, and cost-effectiveness, patients have reservations completing the examination due to embarrassment surrounding the bowel preparation and invasiveness of the procedure.[19] Although FIT screening has lower sensitivity when compared with colonoscopy, it is associated with higher participation rates.[19] Currently, CRC screening is up to date in only 63% to 69% of adults, with rates lower among minority, underinsured, and vulnerable populations.[20] It is important to understand the barriers faced by different populations and strategies to overcome these barriers.

Barriers to Screening

A meta-analysis of 94 studies showed a significant barrier to CRC screening is awareness, including awareness of the disease, reasons to screen asymptomatic individuals, and different screening modalities.[21] In an effort to increase awareness, the use of educational videos and booklets has shown only a small influence in the rates of CRC screening.[21] Patients from a lower socioeconomic status encounter multiple

Table 6
Comparison of recommended colorectal cancer screening guidelines across different organizations

Recommended Colorectal Cancer Screening Guidelines for Average-Risk[a] Adults				
	USPSTF	ACG	ACP	MSTF
Age	50–75 y 76–85 y individualized	50 y except AA start at age 45 y	50–75 y Do not screen if >75 y and life expectancy <10 y	50–75 y except AA start at age 45 y
gFOBT	Annually	Annually	Annually	———
FIT	Annually	Annually	Annually	Annually (Tier 1)
FIT-DNA	Every 1–3 y	Every 3 y	———	Every 3 y (Tier 2)
FS	Every 5 y	Every 5–10 y	Every 5 y	Every 5–10 y (Tier 2)
Colonoscopy	Every 10 y	Every 10 y	Every 10 y	Every 10 y (Tier 1)
FIT-FS combination	———	———	FIT every 3 y and FS every 5 y	———
CT colonography	———	———	———	Every 5 y (Tier 2)

Abbreviation: AA, African American.

[a] Average risk is defined as an asymptomatic individual without a personal history of CRC, polyps, inflammatory bowel disease, suspected hereditary CRC syndrome, or history of radiation to the abdomen or pelvis, and no family history of CRC.

barriers including scheduling, taking time off to screen, and transportation issues.[21] Patients from rural communities attribute financial concerns, sense of embarrassment or violation, decreased awareness, and lack of a provider's recommendation as barriers to CRC screening.[22]

CRC screening rates are low among vulnerable populations, including racial and ethnic minorities.[16] Only 42% of Latino men and 47.5% of Latino women have been appropriately screened according to CRC guidelines.[5] As a result, Latino patients are more likely to be diagnosed with CRC when the disease is more advanced.[5] African Americans are less likely to be screened (55.5% prevalence compared with 61.5% among whites)[23] and have a higher incidence of CRC when compared with white patients.[24] Adams and colleagues found that medical mistrust negatively affected rates of CRC screening in African Americans,[24] whereas shared decision-making improves rates of screening.[16]

Screening interventions to improve CRC screening rates include patient-level, provider-level, and system-level interventions.[23] Patient-level interventions include one-on-one education, client screening reminders, and reducing structural barriers.[23] To improve screening rates, providers need to understand the importance of using culturally appropriate strategies. One-on-one education improves awareness, but it does not always have to come from the provider. Client reminders include letters, emails, postcards, or telephone calls that remind patients they are due or overdue for CRC screening.[23] Client reminders can increase screening rates by 5% to 15%.[23]

Provider-level interventions include chart audits, electronic provider reminders, and training on communicating with low-health-literate patients.[23] Chart audits modestly improve CRC screening by 12.3% to 30%, electronic reminder improve screening rates by 5%, and using trained providers to communicate with low-health-literate patients improves screening by 10% to 15%.[23]

System-level interventions use patient navigators to help patients access screening services. With Latinos, studies show the use of patient navigators improves CRC screening rates.[5] Patient navigators work with patients to better understand the health care system and overcome barriers.[23] Overall use of patient navigators improves screening by 10% to 15% and can increase screen rates by an additional 15% when compared with one-on-one education alone.[23]

Harms of Screening

When deciding which CRC modality to use, risks of harm associated with the screening is an important factor to consider. Providers must consider the false-negative and false-positive results associated with a screening modality along with the potential risk of the screening test itself. Data show that 10% of patients with a negative FIT have CRC or a precancerous lesion.[25] False-negative results may give patients and providers a false reassurance, which in turn could delay CRC diagnosis.[25] Risks factors associated with false-negative FIT screening results include male patients, family history of CRC, patients with elements of the metabolic syndrome (specifically obesity, hyperglycemia, and hypertension), and former or current smokers.[25]

Patients who have a positive FIT screening test are typically referred for additional testing via a colonoscopy. False-positive FIT results carry a risk of harm, as unnecessary invasive testing with colonoscopy is recommended, and patients may experience psychological distress between receiving results of the FIT test and the outcome of the colonoscopy test.[25] Risk factors associated with false-positive FIT testing include use of nonsteroidal antiinflammatory drugs, presence of anal fissure, and use of a proton pump inhibitor.[25]

Colonoscopy has its own set of discomfort and harms. To evaluate the entire colon correctly, patients must do a thorough bowel cleansing. This bowel prep can be embarrassing and uncomfortable for patients, and a poor prep may limit the effectiveness of this screening modality. Colonoscopy carries a higher risk of bowel perforation when compared with other screening modalities and a small risk for splenic injury requiring splenectomy.[9] In addition, when deep sedation is offered, the risk for developing aspiration pneumonitis increases.[9] Colonoscopy carries a greater risk of postprocedural bleeding when compared with other screening modalities, especially related to polypectomy and electrocautery.[9] Flexible sigmoidoscopy when compared with colonoscopy has a lower cost and risk, the bowel preparation is limited, and does not require sedation.[9] A significant potential harm of FS includes missing a proximal colon cancer or precancerous lesion.

SUMMARY

CRC screening for average-risk adults is cost-effective, cost-saving, and should be recommended as part of a preventative approach to patient care. Because there are multiple guidelines without clear concordance in recommendations, providers face a challenge of choosing the best CRC modality for their patients. Most guidelines recommend screening of average-risk adults for CRC beginning at the age of 50 years, except for African Americans who should begin screening at the age of 45 years. Overcoming barriers to CRC screening, thereby increasing the number of individuals who undergo screening is more cost-effective and can save more lives than starting screening at an earlier age.

When deciding which CRC modality to recommend, providers need to take into consideration the sensitivity and specificity of the screening modality, patient preferences, barriers to screening, and the risks versus potential harms of screening. Viable options for CRC screening include annual or biennial stool-based testing, FS every 5 to 10 years, or colonoscopy every 10 years. Improving patient awareness about the different CRC screening modalities and using shared decision-making can help improve the number of patients who undergo screening. Understanding risk factors associated with false-positive and false-negative results is another tool to guide decision-making. Finally, using screening interventions at the patient, provider, and system level can help to improve CRC screening rates.

CLINICS CARE POINTS

- Average-risk adults for CRC screening do not have a personal history of CRC or polyps, a family history of CRC, a personal history of inflammatory bowel disease, a confirmed or suspected hereditary CRC syndrome, or a personal history of radiation to the abdomen/pelvis to treat a previous cancer.

- Average-risk adults should begin CRC screening at the age of 50 years, except African American adults should begin screening at age 45 years.

- Consider stopping CRC screening when older than 75 years in individuals who have a life expectancy less than 10 years.

- CRC screening for average-risk adults is cost-effective, cost saving, and should be recommended as part of a preventative approach to patient care.

DISCLOSURE STATEMENT

The author has nothing to disclose.

REFERENCES

1. American Cancer Society. Cancer Facts & Figures 2020. Atlanta, Ga: American Cancer Society; 2020. Available at: https://www.cancer.org/cancer/colon-rectal-cancer/about/key-statistics.html#: ~ :text=Lifetime%20risk%20of%20colorectal% 20cancer,risk%20for%20developing%20colorectal%20cancer. Updated August 31, 2020. Accessed October 12, 2020.
2. U.S. Cancer Statistics Working Group. U.S. Cancer Statistics data visualizations tool, based on 2019 submission data (1999-2017). U.S. Department of Health and Human Services, Centers for Disease Control and Prevention and National Cancer Institute; 2020. Available at: www.cdc.gov/cancer/dataviz. Accessed October 12, 2020.
3. Centers for Disease Control and Prevention. Use of colorectal cancer screening tests, 2018 behavioral risk factor surveillance system. Available at: https://www.cdc.gov/cancer/colorectal/statistics/use-screening-tests-BRFSS.htm. Updated October 19, 2020. Accessed October 12, 2020.
4. Agency for Healthcare Research and Quality. Total expenditure in millions by condition and event type, United States, 2015. Medical Expenditure Panel Survey.
5. Mojica CM, Parra-Medina D, Vernon S. Interventions promoting colorectal cancer screening among Latino men: a systematic review. Prev Chronic Dis 2018;15: 170281.

6. American Cancer Society. Guidelines for colorectal cancer screening. Available at: https://www.cancer.org/cancer/colon-rectal-cancer/detection-diagnosis-staging/acs-recommendations.html. Accessed October 14, 2020.

7. US Preventive Services Task Force. Colorectal cancer: screening. Available at: https://www.uspreventiveservicestaskforce.org/uspstf/recommendation/colorectal-cancer-screening. Accessed October 14, 2020.

8. Bénard F, Barkun AN, Martel M, et al. Systematic review of colorectal cancer screening guidelines for average-risk adults: summarizing the current global recommendations. WJG 2018;24(1):124–38.

9. Rex DK, Boland RC, Dominitz JA, et al. Colorectal cancer screening: recommendations for physicians and patients from the U.S. multi-society task force on colorectal cancer. G Ital Endod 2017;86(1):18–33.

10. Lin JS, Piper M, Perdue LA, et al. Screening for colorectal cancer: a systematic review for the U.S. preventive services task force. Evidence Synthesis No. 135. AHRQ Publication No. 14-05203-EF-1. Rockville, MD: Agency for Healthcare Research and Quality; 2016.

11. Young GP, Fraser CG, Halloran SP, et al. Guaiac based faecal occult blood testing for colorectal cancer screening: an obsolete strategy? Gut 2012;61(7):959–60.

12. Konrad G. Dietary interventions for fecal occult blood test. Can Fam Physician 2010;56(3):229–38.

13. Fitzpatrick-Lewis D, Ali MU, Warren R, et al. Screening for colorectal cancer: a systematic review and meta-analysis. Clin Colorectal Cancer 2016;15(4):298–313.

14. Scalise P, Mantarro A, Pancrazi F, et al. Computed tomography colonography for the practicing radiologist: a review of current recommendations on methodology and clinical indications. World J Radiol 2016;8(5):472–83.

15. Wang Y, Chen P, Lie R. Advance in plasma SEPT9 gene methylation assay for colorectal cancer early detection. World J Gastrointest Oncol 2018;10(1):15–22.

16. Lee SJ, O'Leary MC, Umble KE, et al. Eliciting vulnerable patients' preferences regarding colorectal cancer screening: a systematic review. Patient Prefer Adherence 2018;12:2267–82.

17. Ran T, Cheng C, Misselwitz B, et al. Cost-effectiveness of colorectal cancer screening strategies: a systematic review. Clin Gastroenterol Hepatol 2019;17(10):1969–81.

18. Ladabaum U, Mannalithara A, Meester RGS, et al. Cost-effectiveness and national effects of initiating colorectal cancer screening for average-risk persons at age 45 years instead of 50 years. Gastroenterology 2019;157(1):137–48.

19. Mendivil J, Appierto M, Aceituno S, et al. Economic evaluations of screening strategies fro the early detection of colorectal cancer in the average-risk population: a systematic literature review. Plos One 2019;14(12):e0227251.

20. Dougherty MK, Brenner AT, Crockett SD, et al. Evaluation of interventions intended to increase colorectal cancer screening rates in the United States. JAMA Intern Med 2018;178(12):1645–58.

21. Honein-AbouHaidar GN, Kastner M, Vuong V, et al. Systematic review and meta-study synthesis of qualitative studies evaluating facilitators and barriers to participation in colorectal cancer screening. Cancer Epidemiol Biomarkers Prev 2016;25(6):907–17.

22. Wang H, Roy S. Barriers of colorectal cancer screening in rural USA: a systematic review. Rural and Remote Health 2019;19:5181.

23. Domingo JLB, Braun KL. Characteristics of effective colorectal cancer screening navigation programs in federally qualified health centers: a systematic review. J Health Care Poor Underserved 2017;28(1):108–26.
24. Adams LB, Richmond J, Corbie-Smith G, et al. Medical mistrust and colorectal cancer screening among African americans: a systematic review. J Community Health 2017;42(5):1044–61.
25. de Klerk CM, Vendrig LM, Bossuyt PM, et al. Participant-related risk factors for false-positive and false-negative fecal immunochemical tests in colorectal cancer screening: systematic review and meta-analysis. Am J Gastroeterol 2018;113: 1778–87.

Irritable Bowel Syndrome-Strategies for Diagnosis and Management

Amy Kassebaum-Ladewski, PA-C, RD, MMS

KEYWORDS

- IBS • Irritable bowel syndrome • Constipation • Diarrhea • Abdominal pain
- Bloating • Distension

KEY POINTS

- Irritable bowel syndrome (IBS) is a chronic relapsing brain-gut disorder characterized by abdominal pain associated with altered defecation.
- IBS is not a diagnosis of exclusion and can be confidently diagnosed by adhering to specific diagnostic criteria and ruling out alarm signs/symptoms, thereby avoiding superfluous diagnostic testing.
- The pathophysiology of IBS continues to evolve, and likely represents a constellation of underlying etiologies.
- Treatment for IBS is not a one-size-fits-all approach and requires personalized dietary, behavioral therapy, and pharmaceutical interventions.

INTRODUCTION

Irritable bowel syndrome (IBS) is a chronic-relapsing brain-gut disorder, also known as a functional gastrointestinal (GI) disorder, characterized by abdominal pain associated with altered defecation. Roughly, 5% to 12% of the US population have symptoms consistent with IBS, making it one of the most common conditions seen in primary care and gastroenterology.[1,2] Women are impacted twice as frequently as men, with peak age of onset occurring between 23 and 54 years.[3] Owing to the biopsychosocial complexity of the disorder, about 25% of patients diagnosed with IBS have sought health care assistance from 5 or more practitioners before a diagnosis is confirmed. Furthermore, demands from debilitated patients and clinician uncertainty lead to superfluous diagnostic testing. These factors result in combined direct and indirect costs exceeding $20 billion per year.[4] Consequently, it is imperative that clinicians make accurate and confident diagnoses and institute appropriate treatment recommendations for these patients. Physician assistants, admired for compassionate and patient-first care, are therefore in a unique

Digestive Health Center, Northwestern Memorial Hospital, 259 E Erie Streey, suite 1600, Chicago, IL 60611, USA
E-mail address: akasseba@nm.org

Physician Assist Clin 6 (2021) 637–653
https://doi.org/10.1016/j.cpha.2021.05.008
2405-7991/21/© 2021 Elsevier Inc. All rights reserved.
physicianassistant.theclinics.com

position to invest the time and counseling required to provide comprehensive care to individuals with IBS.

DISCUSSION
Diagnosing Irritable Bowel Syndrome

IBS is neither a diagnosis of exclusion nor a coverall for a constellation of abdominal and bowel symptoms. A limited evaluation is all that is necessary to rule out an underlying organic disease. If an individual meets ROME IV criteria (**Box 1**) combined with an absence of alarm symptoms (**Box 2**), the pretest probability that a patient has IBS approaches 97% to 98%.[5,6] Furthermore, among patients meeting symptom-based criteria for IBS, the likelihood of missing inflammatory bowel disease (IBD), colorectal cancer, or infectious diarrhea can be as low as 1%, with recommended diagnostic tests rarely identifying organic GI disease.[7]

Box 1
Rome IV diagnostic criteria for IBS[5]

Recurrent abdominal *pain*, on average, ≥1 day per week in the last 3 months, associated with ≥2 of the following:

- Related to defecation
- Change in frequency of stool
- Change in form (appearance) of stool

Criteria should be fulfilled for the last 3 months with symptom onset ≥6 months before the diagnosis

---

Box 2
GI alarm signs and symptoms[6]

Unexplained weight loss

Rectal bleeding or melena

Nocturnal diarrhea

Fevers

Unexplained iron-deficiency anemia

Symptom onset after 50 years of age

Severe or progressively worsening symptoms

Family history of organic GI diseases (colorectal cancer, Celiac disease, or IBD)

There are 4 subtypes of IBS: IBS with diarrhea (IBS-D), IBS with constipation (IBS-C), IBS mixed (IBS-M), and IBS un-subtyped (IBS-U).[8] The Bristol Stool Form Scale (BSFS) is used to standardize stool consistency, with textures ranging from Bristol 1 (hard lumps) to a Bristol 7 (watery) (**Table 1**).[9] IBS-D (35%) is the most common subtype followed by IBS-M (30%), IBS-C (30%), and IBS-U (5%).[2]

Table 1
Defining IBS subtype based on the Bristol Stool Form Scale (BSFS)

	BSFS[9]	IBS Subtypes[5]
Type 1	Separate hard lumps, like nuts (hard to pass)	IBS-C
Type 2	Sausage-shaped but lumpy	Bristol 1–2 $\geq$ 25%
		Bristol 6–7 $\leq$ 25%
Type 3	Like a sausage, but with cracks on the surface	IBS-M
Type 4	Like a sausage or snack, smooth and soft	Bristol 1–2 $\geq$ 25%
Type 5	Soft blobs with clear-cut edges (passed easily)	Bristol 6–7 $\geq$ 25%
Type 6	Fluffy pieces with ragged edges, a mush stool	IBS-D
Type 7	Watery, no solid pieces (entirely liquid)	Bristol 1–2 $\leq$ 25%
		Bristol 6–7 $\geq$ 25%

Pathophysiology

Our understanding of the complex and heterogeneous pathogenesis of IBS continues to evolve. **Box 3**, extrapolated from a clinical review of IBS published in the Journal of American Medical Association, summarizes the primary etiologies of IBS.[10] Like other functional GI disorders, IBS is highly influenced by alterations in the gut-brain axis. The gut-brain axis is a bidirectional communication system between the GI tract and the central nervous system, and is modified by environmental and anatomic factors including the hypothalamus-pituitary axis, limbic system, autonomic nervous system, and endocrine system.[1] More recently, the gut microbiota has emerged as another potential confounder. Alterations to this axis result in changes in intestinal motility, secretion, and sensation.

Box 3
Etiologies of IBS[10]

Host Factors
- Visceral hypersensitivity
- Altered gut-brain interactions
- Dysbiosis
- Increased intestinal permeability
- Gut mucosal immune activation
- Bile acid malabsorption

Environmental Factors
- Early life stressors (abuse, psychosocial stressors)
- Food intolerance
- Antibiotics
- Enteric infection

The biopsychosocial model for gut-brain disorders illustrates the interplay between early life (genetic, environment), psychosocial (life stress, psychological state, coping, social support), and physiologic factors (motility, visceral hypersensitivity, inflammation, food intolerance, infection, altered bacterial flora, increased bile acids), which ultimately results in IBS symptoms and behaviors.[11] In an important epidemiologic study, 60% of women with GI disorders (39% with a functional GI diagnosis) reported a history of adult or childhood sexual or physical abuse, supporting a relationship between stress and gut-brain dysfunction.[12] Furthermore, GI infections are well-known precipitants of postinfectious IBS (PI-IBS). Enteric luminal infections (bacterial, viral, and parasitic) not only induce a proinflammatory response but also result in dysbiosis, changes in neuroendocrine mediators, and an increase in bile acids.[13] The incidence of PI-IBS ranges from 3.7% to 36% and can last up to 6 and 8 years after the acute illness.

Creating a Differential Diagnosis

A detailed medical and surgical history and medication review is necessary to prevent overlooking other primary or secondary sources of constipation and diarrhea. **Boxes 4 and 5** review the differential diagnoses of IBS-C and IBS-D.

Box 4
Differential IBS-C

Chronic idiopathic constipation
- Normal transit constipation
- Slow transit constipation

Medication-induced constipation
- Ex: anticholinergics, bile acid sequestrants, calcium channel blockers, diuretics, iron, narcotics, polypharmacy

Anatomic
- Ex: rectal stricture, rectal prolapse/intussusception, rectocele

Functional dyssynergic defecation

Secondary causes
- Neurogenic (Parkinson's, multiple sclerosis)
- Endocrine (diabetes mellitus, hypothyroidism)
- Malignancy (ovarian cancer)
- Pregnancy

Colonic methanogenic bacterial overgrowth

Differential Diagnosis for IBS-C: Key Disorders to Consider

Functional defecation disorders

Functional defecation disorders (FDDs) represent a class of disorders often overlooked but frequently overlap with IBS-C. They are characterized by dyscoordination of the abdominal wall and pelvic floor musculature. A study by Rao and colleagues discovered that 31% of patients with an FDD experienced constipation since childhood, 29% developed it after an acute event such as pregnancy, trauma, or back injury, and in 40% of cases, no cause could be identified.[14] Alarmingly, physical abuse was reported by 32% of patients, with 22% of reports being sexual abuse, and most were women. These data are supportive of the importance of inquiring about an abuse or trauma history, once trust and rapport have been established. The overlapping nature of FDD with IBS-C is a common reason why patients fail to respond to IBS therapy.

A digital rectal examination identifying high resting sphincter tone and/or paradoxic contraction or an inability to relax the pelvic floor upon bearing down can help support a diagnosis of FDD.[15] If an individual with IBS-C fails initial evidence-based treatments, referral for specialized pelvic floor testing (ie, anorectal manometry and balloon expulsion testing) is recommended.

Box 5
Differential for IBS-D

Functional diarrhea

Medication-induced diarrhea:
- Ex: antibiotics, chemotherapy, colchicine, digoxin or lithium toxicity, immunosuppressants (mycophenolate), proton pump inhibitors, magnesium, metformin, NSAIDs, SSRIs

Microscopic colitis

Celiac disease

Infectious diarrhea

Small intestinal bacterial overgrowth

Inflammatory bowel disease

Bile acid diarrhea

Food intolerance

Carbohydrate malabsorption (lactose intolerance)

Constipation with overflow diarrhea

Differential Diagnosis for IBS-D: Key Disorders to Consider

Inflammatory Bowel Disease

Neglecting to diagnose IBD in a patient presenting with abdominal pain and diarrhea is an understandable concern for clinicians. Alarm signs or symptoms including rectal bleeding, iron deficiency anemia, involuntary weight loss, an acute change in bowel habits, a family history of IBD, and/or the presence of extraintestinal manifestations (unexplained rashes, joint pain) are indications for proceeding with further diagnostic testing. If the pretest probability of having IBD is low and none of the aforementioned alarm signs or symptoms are present, a stool fecal calprotectin and a serum C-reactive protein (CRP) can be checked with normal values essentially ruling out both IBD and the need for endoscopic testing.[16] In a systemic review of 12 studies (N = 2145), serum CRP and fecal calprotectin were compared between adult patients with IBD, IBS, and healthy controls. The results revealed that at a threshold of 40 for fecal calprotectin and 0.5 for CRP, the percentage likelihood of missing IBD in an individual with IBS is about 1%. Lower values were associated with even lower risks. Therefore, a low fecal calprotectin and low CRP in individuals meeting IBS criteria essentially rule out IBD. Notably, fecal calprotectin is more sensitive and specific and is preferred over CRP.

Celiac disease

Physician assistants should have a low threshold for checking for celiac disease, especially in patients who endorse a family or personal history of autoimmune disorders, iron deficiency, infertility, or premature reduced bone density.[17] Although celiac disease is presumed to present with diarrhea, up to 15% of patients with celiac disease may present with constipation. Based on the 2021 American College of Gastroenterology (ACG) clinical guideline for the management of IBS, celiac screening is recommended for all individuals with IBS associated with diarrhea, but there are no specific guidelines for IBS-C, and therefore, the decision to test for celiac disease in patients with constipation should be evaluated on an individual basis.[18] Recommended laboratories include serum transglutaminase IgA levels and a quantitative IgA, to assess for possible total IgA deficiency that could induce false-negative results.

For patients with IBS reporting a positive response to an empiric gluten-free (GF) diet who are resistant to reintroducing gluten for at least 4 to 6 weeks to complete antibody testing, consider offering HLA antigen testing. HLA-DQ2 and HLA-DQ8 are positive in almost all patients with celiac disease.[19] However, roughly 50% of the general population and 90% of first-degree relatives of patients with celiac disease will carry these antigens. Therefore, although negative HLA testing basically excludes celiac disease, a positive test does not confidently confirm the diagnosis. If the test is negative, a symptom response to a GF diet may support a diagnosis of non-celiac gluten or wheat sensitivity.

Small intestinal bacterial overgrowth/intestinal methanogenic overgrowth

Small intestinal bacterial overgrowth (SIBO) is broadly defined as excessive colonic-type bacteria in the small intestine leading to increased carbohydrate fermentation and subsequent gas production.[20] Risk factors for SIBO include abnormalities in anatomy (adhesive disease, small-bowel diverticula, postsurgical anatomic alteration), motility (scleroderma, diabetes mellitus, narcotics), pH (achlorhydria, advanced age), and immunity (IgA deficiency, HIV). The nonspecific presentation of SIBO includes abdominal bloating, flatulence, abdominal pain, and diarrhea, similar to IBS. In severe cases, a patient can experience malabsorption leading to weight loss and malnutrition with deficiencies in fat-soluble vitamins (sparing vitamin K because it is a byproduct of bacterial fermentation), B12, and iron. There is controversy in testing for SIBO in patients diagnosed with IBS, although a recent meta-analysis revealed that patients with IBS were 2.6 and 8.3 times more likely to have a positive test for SIBO as compared with healthy controls using a glucose hydrogen breath test (GHBT) and jejunal aspirate culture, respectively.[21] Patients with IBS-D were more likely to have a positive GHBT as compared with the other subtypes. Testing for SIBO with glucose or lactulose breath tests is simple and safe; however, there is significant heterogeneity in test performance, preparation, indications for testing, and interpretation of results.

Box 6
IBS diagnostic testing

All subtypes[10]
- CBC
- Age-appropriate CRC screening

IBS-D
- CRP or fecal calprotectin
- tTG-IgA + quantitative IgA
- When colonoscopy performed, obtain random biopsies
- RF for SIBO/refractory to treatment, consider carbohydrate breath testing
- Consider infectious work-up (giardia) based on RF and exposures

IBS-M
- CRP or fecal calprotectin
- tTG-IgA + quantitative IgA
- Stool diary
- Consider abdominal plain film to assess for fecal loading
- RF for SIBO/refractory to treatment, consider carbohydrate breath testing

IBS-C
- If severe or medically refractory, refer to specialist for physiologic testing

---

Furthermore, more recent data suggest that intestinal methanogenic overgrowth characterized by elevated methane gas levels produced by colonic archaeal species can influence intestinal motor activity leading to intestinal slowing and constipation.[13] A consensus on hydrogen and methane-based breath testing now considers methane (as a surrogate for excess intestinal colonization with methanogens) as beneficial in the assessment of constipation and IBS-C.[22]

Diagnostic Testing

There is no definitive diagnostic laboratory testing for IBS. See **Box 6** to review specific IBS subtype testing.[10]

Management of Irritable Bowel Syndrome

Dietary interventions for irritable bowel syndrome

Dietary counseling is essential as roughly 70% of individuals with gut-brain disorders report an exacerbation of symptoms from eating certain foods.[23] Many patients have already independently tried and failed diet modification before seeking care. When counseling a patient on diet, recommendations should be individualized to the patient's learning level, openness and readiness for change, comorbid medical and psychosocial conditions, and previous diets already attempted and failed. A prior history or evidence of active disordered eating should be elicited as some diets are contraindicated in these circumstances.

Basic dietary tips

Basic counseling tips for the diet naïve patient can be extrapolated from review of the United Kingdom National Institute for Health and Care Excellence (NICE) guidelines, which advices to avoid or limit caffeine, alcohol, sugar alcohols (ie, sorbitol), high fructose beverages/excessive fruit consumption, and insoluble fibers (bran).[24] In addition, a period of lactose avoidance and reintroduction can help identify lactose intolerance. Avoiding uncooked cruciferous vegetables, onions, and garlic may help reduce gas and bloating. Daily exercise, adequate water intake, quality sleep, relaxation, and structured eating behaviors should also be encouraged.[25–27]

Low-fermentable oligo-, di-, monosaccharide and polyol diet

The low fermentable oligo-, di-, monosaccharide and polyol (FODMAP) diet has gained popularity over the past decade. The diet centers on eliminating short-chain carbohydrates that are poorly absorbable and highly fermentable by gut bacteria.[28] Fermentation of short-chain carbohydrates results in an increased osmotic load, local inflammation, and alterations in colonic motility. The primary sources of FODMAPs include fruits with a high fructose to sucrose ratio (honey, apples, peaches, fruit juice), fructans (wheat, rye, onions, garlic, inulin), lactose (milk, ice cream, cottage cheese, ricotta), sorbitol (apricots, peaches, artificial sweeteners), and raffinose (lentils, cabbage, brussels sprouts, legumes). The diet consists of a proof-of-concept 4 to 6 week elimination phase, followed by a slow reintroduction of food classes, and personalization with intent to maintain a more liberalized and less restrictive version of the diet, if certain foods/food groups are identified as the cause of symptoms. If after 4 to 6 weeks, the diet proves ineffective, it can be completely discontinued. Given the complexity, it is recommended that this process be guided by a well-trained registered dietitian. Data on long-term safety and efficacy are lacking, and a major concern is that the diet may potentially alter small intestinal pH, reduce microbial diversity, and ultimately worsen IBS symptoms.[29]

In a comparison between the low-FODMAP diet to a modified NICE diet (FODMAP foods were not eliminated), both proved equally efficacious in relief of global IBS-D symptoms.[30] However, consumption of a low-FODMAP diet did result in early and significantly reduced rates of abdominal pain and bloating (51% vs 23%). Thus, certain symptoms or symptom profiles may respond better to a particular diet over another.

Gluten-free diet

There is limited data to support a GF diet in IBS; however, many patients endorse improvement in bloating, abdominal pain, and stool consistency when adherent to a GF diet.[31] The response to gluten elimination may not be due to the gluten itself, but the large amount of fructans in wheat products, which also increase colonic fermentation. In addition, wheat flours are abundant in processed foods, and these foods typically contain other IBS triggering additives, such as fructose. Consequently, avoidance of processed foods containing wheat products may contribute to favorable

Table 2
Summary of management therapies for IBS-C

Categories of IBS-C Therapies by MOA		Dosing & Administration	Side-Effects
Soluble fiber	Psyllium[32]	1 tbsp QD, increase slowly as needed up to TID	Bloating/gas
Prosecretory agents	Lubiprostone[33,a]	IBS-C: 8 mcg BID CIC: 25 mcg BID Take with meals	Nausea, diarrhea, headache
Prosecretory agents 5HT4 Agonist	Linaclotide[34,b]	IBS-C: 290 mcg QD CIC: 72 mcg & 145 mcg QD Take at least 30 min before first meal	Diarrhea
	Plecanatide[35,b]	IBS-C & CIC: 3 mg QD Take with or without meals	Diarrhea
	Tegaserod[43,c]	IBS-C: 2 mg QD Take at least 30 min before first meal	Headache, abdominal pain, nausea, diarrhea CI: hx of MI, stroke, TIA, angina, intestinal ischemia, severe renal impairment, severe hepatic impairment
Neuromodulators	SSRIs/TCAs[55]	Start with a low dose and titrate slowly by response, allowing 6–8 wk for maximal response. Continue at the minimum effective dose for at least 6–12 mo	TCAs: dry mouth, dry eyes, arrhythmia, orthostatic hypotension, sexual dysfunction SSRIs: diarrhea, nausea, headache
Psychological therapies	Gut-directed behavioral therapy[56] Hypnotherapy[58]	At least 4 sessions over 10 wk	Poorly reported

[a] Approved for IBS-C in women older than 18 years.
[b] FDA approved for IBS-C.
[c] Approved for IBS-C in women younger than 65 years.

responses. Conversely, a GF diet does not equate to healthy, as it can be stripped of fiber, fortified b vitamins, and folate. If the celiac disease has been ruled out (while eating gluten), and a patient is interested in trying a GF diet or has been responsive to a GF diet in the past, a low gluten diet instead of a strict GF diet should be encouraged.

Treatment of IBS-C

Table 2 includes a summary of supported treatment therapies for IBS-C.

Fiber

The soluble fiber psyllium (ispaghula), is an inexpensive and evidence-based treatment for mild IBS-C symptoms. Psyllium is minimally fermentable thereby reducing gas and bloating, and it retains its gel-forming and water retention properties in the large bowel.[32] Contrarily, insoluble fibers including bran, provide no benefit for IBS symptoms and may exacerbate bloating and abdominal pain. Patients should be advised to aim for a daily total fiber intake of 20 to 30 g, with a focus on soluble fibers. To reduce side-effects of bloating and gas, start psyllium powder at 1 tbsp daily, and titrate as needed and tolerated (see Table 2). It is also important to counsel patients on drinking adequate amounts of water to assist with fiber consumption.

Polyethylene glycol

Polyethylene glycol (PEG) is a safe over-the-counter osmotic laxative. It is effective in treating constipation, although, studies have shown no benefit for reducing abdominal symptoms in patients with IBS.[18] For this reason, current guidelines suggest against the use of PEG for treating global IBS symptoms.

Prosecretory Agents: Lubiprostone, Linaclotide, Plecanatide

Currently, there are three secretagogues FDA approved for IBS-C: lubiprostone, linaclotide, and plecanatide. As a class, secretagogues are safe therapies to initiate as first-line agents. They have minimal systemic absorption, no drug-drug interactions, and do not require dose adjustments in patients with kidney or liver disease.[33–35] All three agents have proven effective for treating global and individual abdominal and bowel symptoms for long-term management. Therefore, secretagogues are designed to be tried before referring to a gastroenterologist. Secretagogues continue to have improved insurance coverage and can be an affordable option.

Chloride channel 2 (ClC-2) protein agonist: lubiprostone

Lubiprostone, a prostaglandin derivative, acts directly on (ClC-2) receptors in the intestinal mucosa stimulating chloride and fluid secretion, and secondary motility.[36] In 2007, lubiprostone was the first secretagogue FDA approved for IBS-C in adult women at a dose of 8 mcg twice daily.[33] In two large randomized trials, a pooled analysis showed that 18% (10% in placebo) of patients receiving lubiprostone 8 mcg twice daily $\times$ 12 weeks experienced global symptom improvement. The primary efficacy endpoint used a 7-point Likert scale (from significantly relieved to significantly worse) and responders were defined as those who rated their IBS symptoms as being at least moderately relieved for all 4 weeks of the month or significantly relieved for at least 2 weeks of the month for 2 of 3 months of the study.[36] Efficacy and safety were sustained for 9 to 13 months in an open-label extension trial.[37] The primary side-effect is nausea, which is dose-dependent (8 mcg twice daily—8%, 24 mcg twice daily—29%) and may be mitigated by taking lubiprostone with meals.[33] Lubiprostone comes in an 8 mcg and 24 mcg dose, and the rate of nausea is dose-dependent. The 8 mcg dose is FDA approved for IBS-D.

Guanylate cyclase C agonists: linaclotide, plecanatide

Guanylate cyclase C (GC-C) agonists, as their names imply, activate GC-C receptors embedded in the mucosal surfaces of the GI tract resulting in increased luminal fluid secretion and accelerated transit.[38] Preclinical and animal studies have also indicated that agonism of GC-C receptors reduces stimulation of visceral afferent neurons, and this pathway is thought to be an important mechanism in explaining the pain-reducing benefits associated with these agents.[39]

Linaclotide

Linaclotide was FDA approved in 2012 for treating IBS-C and CIC.[34] In two phase 3 trials, consumption of 290 mcg of linaclotide once-daily resulted in a 33% improvement in IBS-C symptoms at 12 weeks in both studies compared with 14% and 21% responses with placebo in each of the two individuals studies, respectively.[40] The primary efficacy endpoint was the percentage of overall responders (patients reporting $\geq$30% reduction from baseline in worst abdominal pain plus an increase of $\geq$1 complete spontaneous bowel movement per week from baseline in the same week for $\geq$6 of 12 treatment weeks). Diarrhea was the most common adverse event (AE) occurring in 20% of those taking linaclotide 290 mcg versus 2.5% of those consuming placebo. Only 2% of patients experienced severe diarrhea. Linaclotide comes in three doses, 72 mcg, 145 mcg, and 290 mcg, with the rate of diarrhea being dose-dependent, and should be dosed at least 30 min before the first meal to mitigate the side-effect of diarrhea.[34] The 290 mcg dose is FDA approved for IBS-D.

Plectanatide

Plecanatide was FDA approved in 2017 for treatment of IBS-C and CIC.[35] Plecanatide differs from linaclotide in that it mimics the effects of the naturally occurring GC-C agonist, uroguanylin.[41] Uroguanylin, a pH-dependent peptide secreted by the enterochromaffin cells in the small intestine in response to a meal, actives GC-C receptors predominately in the small bowel and less in the colon, thereby potentially reducing the likelihood of diarrhea.

Statistically significant improvements in IBS-C–related symptoms were identified in two large phase 3, 12-week trials. The primary endpoint in these studies was identical to those used in the linaclotide trials. Overall response rates to a 3 mg daily dose of plecanatide were 30% compared to 18% with placebo in study 1 and 21% compared to 14% in study 2.[42] The most common AE was diarrhea occurring in 4.3% of those treated with plecanatide compared with 1% of individuals receiving placebo. Severe diarrhea occurred in less than 1% of patients. Plecanatide only comes in one dose, 3 mg, and can be taken with or without food.[35]

5HT4 receptor agonist: tegaserod

Tegaserod, a 5-hydroxytryptamine-4 (5-HT4) agonist, was reapproved by the FDA in 2019 for treating women with IBS-C aged less than 65 years with no hx of cardiovascular ischemic events.[43] Tegaserod, selective for the type 4 serotonin receptors in the gut, stimulates intestinal secretion, which directly induces colonic motility and decreases visceral sensitivity. Its efficacy is supported by four 12-week randomized, placebo-controlled trials assessing women with IBS aged less than 65 years without cardiovascular ischemic events who received tegaserod 6 mg twice daily or placebo (N = 2752).[44] Using the Subjective Global Assessment (SGA), responders were defined as rating themselves "considerably" or "completely" relieved $\geq$50% of the time or at least "somewhat relieved" 100% of the time over the first 4 weeks and the last 4 weeks of the 12-week studies. At 4 weeks, 35% of patients receiving tegaserod were responders (21% in placebo) and over the last 4 weeks, 44% were

Table 3
Summary of management therapies for IBS-D

Categories of IBS-D Therapies by MOA		Dosing & Administration	Adverse Effects
Modulation of gut flora	Rifaximin[47,a]	550 mg TID × 14 d w/option for 2 retreatments Take with or without food	Headache, nausea, abdominal pain
	Low-FODMAP diet[28]	6-wk elimination with slow reintroduction	Possible impact on gut microbiome
Bile acid sequestrants	Cholestyramine, colestid, colesevelam[52]	BID before meals May alter absorption of some medications— take other medications 1 h before or 4 h after	Constipation
Opioid receptor modulator	Eluxadoline[50,a]	100 mg BID 75 mg BID (intolerant of 100 mg, receiving OATP1B1 inhibitors, mild to moderate hepatic impairment) Take with food	Constipation, nausea, abdominal pain, sphincter of Oddi spasm, pancreatitis
Antispasmodic	Peppermint oil[53,54]	2 capsules TID before meals, reduce to lowest effective dose Take 30 to 90 min before meals	Heartburn, dyspepsia
Neuromodulators/ Behavioral therapy	See Table 2	See Table 2	See Table 2

[a] FDA approved for IBS-D.

responders (36.5% in placebo). The responder rate of combined pooled responders at 4 and 12 weeks was not included with the current available data.

The most common side-effects are headaches (14% vs 10% in placebo), abdominal pain (11% vs 10%), nausea (8% vs 7%), and diarrhea (8% vs 3%).[43] Tegaserod should not be used in patients with advanced kidney and liver disease. Tegaserod is dosed at 6 mg twice per day at least 30 min before meals.

Treatment of IBS-D

Table 3 includes a summary of supported treatment therapies for IBS-D.

Rifaximin

FDA approved in 2015 for treatment of IBS-D, rifaximin is an oral, nonsystemic bactericidal antibiotic that works to modulate microbiota.[45] It is the most studied drug in IBS-D, and has shown significant benefit, especially in the setting of postinfectious IBS-D. In 2 large double-blind placebo-controlled trials designed to assess the primary endpoint of adequate relief of pain and stool consistency for at least 2 of the first 4 weeks after treatment, 47% of patients in trials 1 and 2 responded compared with 39% and 36% in the placebo group.[46] The drug is well tolerated with minimal systemic absorption (0.4%).[45] The most common adverse reactions in RCTs with rifaximin were nausea (3% vs 2% in placebo) and an increase in alanine transferase (2% vs 1%).[47] Rifaximin is contraindicated in patients with a known hypersensitivity to it and rifampin. In RCTs, there was only one case of C-diff diarrhea, which occurred in a patient who had recently been treated with a cephalosporin for a urinary tract infection. Rifaximin may affect warfarin activity, but is not contraindicated, and INR levels should be monitored more closely. Rifaximin is dosed at 550 mg 3 times per day for 14 days with an option for 2 retreatments.

Eluxadoline

Eluxadoline is a mixed opioid receptor agonist and antagonist, which modulates motility and pain. It was FDA approved in 2015 for treatment of IBS-D in adults. In 2 randomized, double-blind, placebo-controlled trials of adult patients with IBS-D (N = 2427), there was a significantly greater proportion of eluxadoline patients who experienced improvements in pain and diarrhea (22.7% vs 10.3% in placebo), and this response was sustained over 12 weeks.[48]

The primary endpoint was defined as a ≥30% daily reduction in pain compared with baseline combined with a BSFS to less than 5 on the same day for at least 50% of days within the 12-week treatment period. In a follow-up study assessing patients with IBS-D who had subjectively failed to respond to loperamide in the previous 12 months, patients receiving eluxadoline experienced significant improvements in global IBS-D symptoms (22.7% vs 10.3% in placebo).[49] Eluxadoline is dosed at 100 mg twice per day with meals or 75 mg twice per day in those who do not tolerate the 100 mg dose, take OATP1B1 inhibitors, or have mild to moderate hepatic impairment.[50] Primary side-effects include constipation (8.6%), nausea (7.5%), and abdominal pain (7.2%). Eluxadoline is contraindicated in patients who do not have a gallbladder or have bile duct obstruction, sphincter of Oddi dysfunction, a history of pancreatitis, severe liver impairment, severe constipation, and/or consume greater than 3 alcohol drinks per day.

Bile acid sequestrants

A meta-analysis of 6 studies reporting on IBS-D symptoms revealed that bile acid malabsorption was evident in 16.9% to 35.3% of the individuals diagnosed with IBS-D; however, quality randomized controlled trials of use of bile acid sequestrants (BAS) to treat IBS-D are limited.[51] Therefore, BAS are not FDA approved for IBS-D, but are a therapy to consider for the management of diarrhea. BAS can interfere with the absorption of certain medications (ie, levothyroxine) and fat-soluble vitamins, and should be administered at least 4 hours apart.[52] A pharmacist can assist in assessing medication interactions and administration of BAS. Patients should be cautioned on the risk for rebound constipation.

Complementary Therapies for IBS-C and IBS-D

Peppermint oil

Peppermint oil has shown benefit in improving IBS symptoms through its antispasmodic, anti-inflammatory, antibacterial, and serotonergic antagonistic properties in the digestive tract.[53] Given minimal adverse effects, peppermint oil is a safe therapy for IBS patients looking for a natural remedy, although overall data are weak and limited. A well-known side-effect of peppermint oil is heartburn; however, an over-the-counter triple-coated microspherical formulation may minimize this effect.[54] This formulation was studied in an RCT of patients with IBS-D and IBS-M (N = 72) with statistically significant improvements in IBS symptoms noted at 4 weeks (40% compared with 25% in placebo).

Probiotics

Most clinicians and patients can attest to receiving mixed messages regarding the use of probiotics in patients with IBS. The 2021 ACG guideline on IBS recommends against the use of probiotics for treating IBS.[18] Previously published studies vary in bias, heterogenicity, strain types and dosing, and clinical outcomes, which reduces generalizability. The types, combinations, formulations, manufacturing, and shelf lives of probiotics are other variables that convolute the probiotic picture.

Neuromodulators for irritable bowel syndrome

A meta-analysis of 16 RCTs demonstrated that tricyclic antidepressants (TCAs) and selective serotonin reuptake inhibitors (SSRIs) reduce global IBS symptoms and abdominal pain in IBS patients.[55] Specifically, TCAs are the best-studied antidepressants in IBS. When deciding between starting a TCA versus SSRI, a clinician must consider specific symptoms. TCAs have robust neuromodulating effects and are better than SSRIs for pain management. The anticholinergic properties of TCAs, known to slow motility, are well suited for IBS-D. SSRIs, known to be more effective at managing anxiety, can be considered in a patient with concomitant anxiety, especially if anxiety is a known driver of IBS symptoms. Stimulation of serotonin receptors may also make these a more appropriate choice in individuals with IBS-C.

Gut-directed behavioral therapy

There is a dearth of evidence supporting gut-directed behavioral interventions as an adjunct therapy for functional GI disorders, especially IBS.[56] Cognitive behavioral therapy (CBT) represents the most widely studied psychotherapy for IBS. A meta-analyses from 2014 found that gut-directed CBT is highly effective in improving bowel symptoms, quality of life, and psychological distress, and that these effects persist beyond the treatment phase and into long-term follow-up. Studies have found that as little as 4 sessions over 10 weeks can be effective in improving IBS symptoms.[57] In areas where specialized gut-directed behavioral psychologists are not available, CBT may also be offered via telehealth or Internet-based protocols.[56]

Gut-directed hypnotherapy is also an effective behavioral intervention, especially for IBS-related pain and for patients who have already attempted gut-directed CBT.[58] Treatment involves 7 to 12 weekly sessions in which the patient learns to achieve a deepened hypnotic state and are then led through a series of scripted, gut-focused imageries with hypnotic suggestions in each session. Hypnotherapy has been shown to have long-term benefits, with 83% of responders in one study maintaining treatment benefits for 1 to 5 years after the course of treatment.[59] Hypnotherapy should be avoided in patients with a history of trauma and post-traumatic stress disorder.

SUMMARY

IBS is a highly prevalent chronic-relapsing gut-brain disorder, which significantly impacts the quality of life. Through a detailed history, assessment for alarm symptoms and evaluation of basic laboratory parameters, a confident diagnosis can be made without extensive testing. As our understanding of pathophysiology of IBS evolves, it is clear that this is not a simple cause-and-effect disorder but one that reflects the interplay between multiple biopsychosocial factors. To promote patient-first care, physician assistants must establish rapport, express empathy, allocate time for counseling and education, and set expectations on outcomes. A detailed understanding of dietary, pharmacologic, and behavioral interventions is essential to provide comprehensive care for patients with IBS.

CLINICS CARE POINTS

- Roughly, 12% of the US adult population suffers with IBS symptoms, yet many never receive a formal diagnosis.

- A confident diagnosis of IBS can be made with basic laboratory testing.
- A diagnosis of IBS does not require a colonoscopy unless the patient is due for a screening colonoscopy or the patient presents with alarm signs and symptoms.
- In one study, 39% of patients with functional GI disorders reported a history of adult or childhood sexual or physical abuse.
- Postinfectious IBS is a well-supported etiology of IBS and can last up to 8 years after the acute illness.
- 70% of patients with functional Gi disorders report an exacerbation of symptoms from eating certain foods.
- The low-FODMAP is an elimination and reintroduction diet and should be managed by an experienced registered dietitian.
- PEG3350 is good for constipation but does not address the global symptoms of IBS, including bloating and pain.
- Prescription secretagogue therapy (lubiprostone, linaclotide, plectanatide) are safe and effective long-term therapies to prescribe for a majority of patients with IBS-C.
- Rifaximin is a safe and effective nonsystemically absorbed antibiotic FDA approved for the treatment of IBS-D.
- In IBS-D patients who have failed OTC loperamide, eluxadoline provided statistically significant improvement in pain and diarrhea.
- In 2018, the American College of Gastroenterology provided a weak recommendation for the use of probiotics to treat IBS symptoms given the low quality of evidence.
- Gut-directed cognitive behavioral therapy is highly effective in improving bowel symptoms, quality of life, and psychological distress.

DISCLOSURE

The author is a consultant for Ironwood pharmaceuticals the maker of linaclotide, Salix pharmaceuticals the maker of plecanatide and rifaximin, and Alfasigma pharmaceuticals the maker of tegaserod.

REFERENCES

1. Lovell RM, Ford AC. Global prevalence of and risk factors for irritable bowel syndrome: a meta-analysis. Clin Gastroenterol Hepatol 2012;10(7):712–21.
2. Palsson OS, Whitehead W, Törnblom H, et al. Prevalence of Rome IV Functional Bowel Disorders Among Adults in the United States, Canada, and the United Kingdom. Gastroenterology 2020;158:1262–73.
3. Hungin AP, Chang L, Locke GR, et al. Irritable bowel syndrome in the United States: prevalence, symptom patterns and impact. Aliment Pharmacol Ther 2005;21:1365–75.
4. Agarwal N, Spiegel BM. The effect of irritable bowel syndrome on health-related quality of life and health care expenditures. Gastroenterol Clin North Am 2011; 40:11–9.
5. Lacy BE, Patel NK. Rome Criteria and a Diagnostic Approach to Irritable Bowel Syndrome. J Clin Med 2017;6(11):99.
6. Vanner SJ, Depew WT, Paterson WG, et al. Predictive Value of the Rome Criteria for Diagnosing the Irritable Bowel Syndrome. Am J Gastroenterol 1999;94(10): 2912–7.

7. Cash BD, Schoenfeld P, Chey W. The Utility of Diagnostic Tests in Irritable Bowel Syndrome Patients: A Systematic Review. Am J Gastroenterol 2002;97(11): 2812–9.

8. Lacy BE, Mearin F, Chang e L, et al. Bowel Disorders. Gastroenterology 2016; 150:1393–407.

9. Lewis SJ, Heaton KW. Stool form scale as a useful guide to intestinal transit time. Scand J Gastroenterol 1997;32:920–4.

10. Chey WD, Kurlander J, Eswaran S. Irritable Bowel Syndrome: A Clinical Review. J Am Med Assoc 2015;313(9):949–58.

11. Tanaka Y, Kanazawa M, Fukudo S, et al. Biopsychosocial model of irritable bowel syndrome. J Neurogastroenterol Motil 2011;17(2):131–9.

12. Drossman DA. Abuse, trauma, and GI illness: Is there a link? Am J Gastroenterol 2011;106(1):14–25.

13. Pimentel M, Lembo A. Microbiome and its Role in Irritable Bowel Syndrome. Dig Dis Sci 2020;65(3):829–39.

14. Rao SS, Tuteja AK, Vellema T, et al. Dyssynergic defecation: demographics, symptoms, stool patterns, and quality of life. J Clin Gastroenterol 2004;38(8): 680–5.

15. Rao SS. Dyssynergic Defecation and Biofeedback Therapy. Gastroenterol Clin North Am 2008;37(3):569–86.

16. Menees SB, Powell C, Kurlander J, et al. A meta-analysis of the utility of C-reactive protein, erythrocyte sedimentation rate, fecal calprotectin, and fecal lactoferrin to exclude inflammatory bowel disease in adults with IBS. Am J Gastroenterol 2015;110:444–54.

17. Green HR. The Many Faces of Celiac Disease: Clinical Presentation of Celiac Disease in the Adult Population. Gastroenterol 2005;128:74–8.

18. Lacy BE, Pimentel M, Brenner DM, et al. ACG Clinical Guideline: Management of Irritable Bowel Syndrome. Am J Gastroenterol 2021;116(1):17–44.

19. Cecilio LA, Bonatto MW. The prevalence of HLA DQ2 and DQ8 in patients with celiac disease, in family and in general population. Arq Bras Cir Dig 2015; 28(3):183–5.

20. Grace E, Shaw C, Whelan K, et al. Review article: small intestinal bacterial overgrowth–prevalence, clinical features, current and developing diagnostic tests, and treatment. Aliment Pharmacol Ther 2013;38(7):674–88.

21. Shah A, Talley NJ, Jones M, et al. Small Intestinal Bacterial Overgrowth in Irritable Bowel Syndrome: A Systematic Review and Meta-Analysis of Case-Control Studies. Am J Gastroenterol 2020;115(2):190–201.

22. Rezaie A, Buresi M, Lembo A, et al. Hydrogen and Methane-Based Breath Testing in Gastrointestinal Disorders: The North American Consensus. Am J Gastroenterol 2017;112(5):775–84.

23. James SC, et al. Gut Microbial Metabolites and Biochemical Pathways Involved in Irritable Bowel Syndrome: Effects of Diet and Nutrition on the Microbiome. J Nutr 2019;00:1–10.

24. Hookway C, Buckner S, Crosland P, et al. Irritable bowel syndrome in adults in primary care: Summary of updated NICE guidance. BMJ 2015;25:350–h701.

25. Zhou C, Zhao E, Li Y, et al. Exercise therapy of patients with irritable bowel syndrome: A systematic review of randomized controlled trials. Neurogastroenterol Motil 2019;31(2):e13461.

26. Patel A, Hasak S, Cassell B, et al. Effects of disturbed sleep on gastrointestinal and somatic pain symptoms in irritable bowel syndrome. Aliment Pharmacol Ther 2016;44(3):246–58.

27. Keefer A, Blanchard E. The effects of relaxation response meditation on the symptoms of irritable bowel syndrome: results of a controlled treatment study. Behav Res Ther 2001;39(7):801–11.
28. Whelan K, Martin L, Staudacher H, et al. The low FODMAP diet in the management of irritable bowel syndrome: an evidence-based review of FODMAP restriction, reintroduction and personalisation in clinical practice. J Hum Nutr Diet 2018; 31:239–55.
29. Hill P, Muir J, Gibson P. Controversies and recent developments of the low-FODMAP diet. Gastroenterol Hepatol NY 2017;13:36–45.
30. Eswaran S, Chey W, Han-Markey T, et al. Am J Gastroenterol. A Randomized Controlled Trial Comparing the Low FODMAP Diet vs. Modified NICE Guidel US Adults IBS-D 2016;111:1824–32.
31. Biesiekeierski J, Newnham E, Irving P, et al. Gluten causes gastrointestinal symptoms in subjects without celiac disease: a double-blind randomized placebo controlled trial. Am J Gastroenterol 2011;106:508–14.
32. Bijkerk C, Wit N, Muris J, et al. Soluble or insoluble fibre in irritable bowel syndrome in primary care? Randomised placebo controlled trial. BMJ 2009;339: b3154.
33. Amitiza (lubiprostone) [package insert]. Bedminster, NJ: Sucampo Pharma Americas, LLC; 2019.
34. Linzess (linaclotide) [package insert]. Cambridge, MA: Ironwood Pharmaceuticals, Inc.; 2018.
35. Trulance (plecanatide) [package insert]. Bridgewater, NJ: Salix Pharmaceuticals, Inc.; 2020.
36. Drossman D, Chey W, Johanson J, et al. Clinical trial: lubiprostone in patients with constipation-associated irritable bowel syndrome – results of two randomized, placebo-controlled studies. Aliment Pharmacol Ther 2009;29:329–41.
37. Chey W, Drossman D, Johanson J, et al. Safety and patient outcomes with lubiprostone for up to 52 weeks in patients with irritable bowel syndrome with constipation. Aliment Pharmacol Ther 2012;35:587–99.
38. Busby R, Bryant A, Bartolini W, et al. Linaclotide, through activation of guanylate cyclase C, acts locally in the gastrointestinal tract to elicit enhanced intestinal secretion and transit. Eur J Pharmacol 2010;649:328–35.
39. Castro J, Harrington A, Hughes P, et al. Linaclotide inhibits colonic nociceptors and relieves abdominal pain via guanylate cyclase-C and extracellular cyclic guanosine 3',5'-monophosphate. Gastroenterol 2013;145:1334–46.
40. Chey W. Linaclotide for Irritable Bowel Syndrome With Constipation: A 26-Week, Randomized, Double-blind, Placebo-Controlled Trial to Evaluate Efficacy and Safety. Am J Gastroenterol 2012;107:1702–12.
41. Rao S. Plecanatide: a new guanylate cyclase agonist for the treatment of chronic idiopathic constipation. Therap Adv Gastroenterol 2018;11. 1756284818777945.
42. Brenner D, Fogel R, Dorn S, et al. Efficacy, safety, and tolerability of plecanatide in patients with irritable bowel syndrome with constipation: results of two phase 3 randomized clinical trials. Am J Gastroenterol 2018;113(5):735–45.
43. ZELNORM (tegaserod) [package insert]. Covington, LA: Alfasigma USA, Inc; 2020.
44. Shah E, Lacy B, Chey W, et al. Efficacy of Tegaserod For Treating Irritable Bowel Syndrome With Constipation in Women <65 Years of Age Without Cardiovascular Risk Factors: A Pooled Analysis of 4 Clinical Trials. Poster presented at American Colelge of Gastroenterology Virtual Annu Meet; October 23-28, 2020; Nashville, TN.

45. Shayto R, Mrad R, Sharara A. Use of rifaximin in gastrointestinal and liver diseases. World J Gastroenterol 2016;22(29):6638–51.
46. Pimentel M, Lembo A, Chey W, et al. Rifaximin Therapy for Patients with Irritable Bowel Syndrome without Constipation. N Engl J Med 2011;364:22–32.
47. Xifaxan (rifaximin) [package insert]. Bridgewater, NJ: Valeant Pharmacueticals North America LLC; 2020.
48. Lembo A, Lacy B, Zuckerman M, et al. Eluxadoline for irritable bowel syndrome with diarrhea. N Engl J Med 2016;374:242–53.
49. Brenner D, Sayuk G, Gutman C, et al. Efficacy and Safety of Eluxadoline in Patients WITH Irritable Bowel Syndrome With Diarrhea Who Report Inadequate Symptom Control With Loperamide: RELIEF Phase 4 Study. Am J Gastroenterol 2019;114(9):1502–11.
50. Viberzi (eluxadoline) [package insert]. Madison, NJ: Allergan USA, Inc.; 2020.
51. Slattery S, Niaz O, Aziz Q, et al. Systematic review with meta-analysis: the prevalence of bile acid malabsorption in the irritable bowel syndrome with diarrhoea. Aliment Pharmacol Ther 2015;42(1):3–11.
52. Welchol (colesevelam) [package insert]. Basking Ridge, NJ: Daiichi Sankyo, Inc; 2019.
53. Khanna R, MacDonald J, Levesque B. Peppermint oil for the treatment of irritable bowel syndrome: a systematic review and meta-analysis. J Clin Gastroenterol 2014;48(6):505–12.
54. Cash B, Estein M, Shah S. A Novel Delivery System of Peppermint Oil is an Effective Therapy for Irritable Bowel Syndrome Symptoms. Dig Dis Sci 2016;61: 560–71.
55. Ford A, Quigley E, Lacy B, et al. Effect of antidepressants and psychological therapies, including hypnotherapy, in irritable bowel syndrome: systemic review of meta-analysis. Am J Gastroenterol 2014;109:1350–65.
56. Li L, Xiong L, Zhang S, et al. Cognitive-behavioral therapy for irritable bowel syndrome: a meta-analysis. J Psychosom Res 2014;77:1–12.
57. Lackner J, Gudleski G, Keefer L, et al. Rapid response to cognitive behavior therapy predicts treatment outcome in patients with irritable bowel syndrome. Clin Gastroenterol Hepatol 2010;8:426–32.
58. Lowén M, Mayer E, Sjöberg M, et al. Effect of hypnotherapy and educational intervention on brain response to visceral stimulus in the irritable bowel syndrome. Aliment Pharmacol Ther 2013;37:1184–97.
59. Gonsalkorale W, Miller V, Afzal A, et al. Long-term benefits of hypnotherapy for irritable bowel syndrome. Gut 2003;52:1623–9.

Inflammatory Bowel Disease: Managing Complex Patients

Paula Miksa, DMS, EdS, MHS, PA-C[a],*,
Shane Ryan Apperley, MSc, PGCert PA-R[b]

KEYWORDS

- Inflammatory bowel disease • Crohn disease • Ulcerative colitis
- Managing complex patients with IBD

KEY POINTS

- An overview of inflammatory bowel disease (IBD) and its two main subtypes, Crohn disease (CD) and ulcerative colitis (UC).
- What are the treatment choices and goals of treatment of patients with CD and UC?
- What makes the management of all patients with IBD "complex"?
- How do we manage special patient groups, namely children, the elderly, and women who are pregnant or breastfeeding?

BACKGROUND

Inflammatory bowel disease is a complex inflammatory disorder involving the gastrointestinal (GI) tract. The disorder varies in location and severity among patients and may be accompanied by extraintestinal manifestations (EM). IBD is classified as either Crohn disease (CD) or ulcerative colitis (UC).

OVERVIEW OF CROHN DISEASE AND ULCERATIVE COLITIS

CD can be found at any location in the GI tract, from the mouth to the anus, whereas UC is limited to the large intestine. Symptoms commonly seen in CD are abdominal pain, diarrhea, and weight loss.[1,2] CD differs from UC histologically due to the involvement of multiple layers of the GI tract, referred to as transmural inflammation. Symptoms correlate with disease location and vary among patients. Physical examination findings can vary from entirely normal to significantly abnormal depending on the

[a] Doctor of Medical Science (DMS) Program, Lincoln Memorial University, 6965 Cumberland Gap Parkway, Harrogate, TN 37752, USA; [b] PA Program, Lincoln Memorial University, 6965 Cumberland Gap Parkway, Harrogate, TN 37752, USA
* Corresponding author.
E-mail address: Paula.Miksa@LMUnet.edu

Physician Assist Clin 6 (2021) 655–665
https://doi.org/10.1016/j.cpha.2021.05.009
2405-7991/21/© 2021 Elsevier Inc. All rights reserved.

physicianassistant.theclinics.com

amount of inflammation and irritation at the time of examination.[1] Owing to the malabsorptive nature of CD, it is common for patients to have nutritional deficiencies. Patients also commonly develop leukocytosis, anemia, and in severe flare-ups, hypoalbuminemia. Clinicians may also order inflammatory markers, namely, C-reactive protein (CRP), erythrocyte sedimentation rate, fecal calprotectin, and quantitative fecal lactoferrin to monitor for signs of remission.[2]

UC generally presents with symptoms of abdominal pain and bloody diarrhea due to its location in the lining of the large intestine. Because UC involves the rectum, there may also be associated symptoms of tenesmus, urgency, rectal pain, and fecal incontinence. As with CD, the severity of symptoms is related to the severity of disease with physical examination often being normal in patients with mild disease.[1,2] In patients with UC with severe symptoms, complications can include perforation or megacolon, especially if the patient was recently diagnosed with UC. Clinicians can order laboratory testing to help determine the severity of disease or a flare. Currently there is no validated or consensus definition on what constitutes mild, moderate, or severe disease; therefore, it is necessary for a clinician to quantify these definitions based on their patients and experience.[1]

CAUSE AND RISK FACTORS

The exact cause of IBD is unknown; however, research has shown that both genetic and environmental factors play a role. First-degree relatives have an increased risk of IBD, and offspring have a higher risk if both parents are affected.[1,2] Cigarette smoking is a risk factor for CD, and conversely, protective against UC. Diet is also associated with the pathogenesis and flare-ups of both CD and UC.[3] IBD is more prevalent in developed countries, especially those in the northern hemisphere, which may suggest that a lack of vitamin D is involved.[1,2]

Patients with IBD are at increased risk for vaccine-preventable illnesses including seasonal influenza. One explanation for this is that vaccines are underutilized in this patient population. Women with IBD, especially those with CD and/or on immunosuppressive therapy, are at an increased risk for developing cervical dysplasia. These patients should therefore undergo Papanicolaou testing annually, as well as receive the human papillomavirus vaccination. Patients with IBD are also at increased risk for developing cancers of the digestive tract, hepatobiliary system, and skin (both melanoma and nonmelanoma). All patients with IBD should therefore be versed on appropriate UV protection and undergo surveillance colonoscopy eight years after diagnosis and every one to two years thereafter.[1]

EXTRAINTESTINAL MANIFESTATIONS

EM affect more than one-third of patients with IBD. Patients with UC with extensive colitis or pancolitis (UC that affects the entire large intestine), and patients with CD that involves the colon, are most affected. EM may occur independently of disease activity, and in some cases, represent the first sign of disease. The musculoskeletal, integumentary, and ocular systems are the most frequently affected systems.[2] Peripheral arthritis, which presents as red, hot, swollen joints, is the most common musculoskeletal EM of IBD. The most commonly occurring dermatologic EM are erythema nodosum (single or multiple tender nodules on the extensor surfaces of the lower extremities) and pyoderma gangrenosum (a papule that rapidly develops into an ulcer with undermined and violaceous borders). Ocular EM include uveitis (headache, blurred vision, and photophobia, an ocular emergency requiring prompt referral to an ophthalmologist) and episcleritis (inflammation of the sclera and conjunctiva), which is most common. Five percent of patients with IBD also develop primary scle-rosing cholangitis (a chronic liver disease characterized by a progressive course of cholestasis with inflammation and fibrosis of the intrahepatic and extrahepatic bile ducts).[1,2]

DIAGNOSIS

As IBD is a disease that can occur anywhere in the GI tract, visualization is required to make a definitive diagnosis. For UC, this is done by colonoscopy and biopsy. Patients who have CD may require additional diagnostic tests. These tests include computed tomography, magnetic resonance enterography, capsule endoscopy, or deep entero-scopy, depending on the location and extent of disease. All patients should undergo a stool examination before diagnosis of UC or CD to exclude infectious colitis.[1,2,4]

In UC, inflammation begins at the rectum and extends proximally. Mucosal edema, erythema, and loss of normal vascular pattern of the intestinal lining is seen in mild UC. Granularity, friability, ulceration, and bleeding are seen in more significant disease. Histologically, altered crypt architecture with shortened, branched crypts in addition to acute and chronic inflammation of the lamina propria is seen.[1,2] In CD, the nature of the inflammation may vary depending on the location of the disease. A patient may have superficial aphthous ulcers of the mouth or deep ulcers of the GI tract with a classic cobblestone appearance.[1,2] CD may appear histologically as patchy transmural inflammation.

There is a small subset (10%–15%) of patients diagnosed with IBD who cannot be categorized as either UC or CD. These patients have a diagnosis of indeterminate co-litis. Serologic tests are an option for these patients; however, these tests are expen-sive, relatively insensitive, and nonspecific.[1]

TREATMENT

The two main goals of IBD therapy are to (1) induce and maintain remission and (2) to prevent disease and treatment-related complications.[1] UC and CD are complex dis-eases, typically requiring complex therapeutic regimes.

CHOICE OF THERAPY

Therapy may involve lifestyle modifications (ie, diet), medical management, and/or surgical intervention.[5] Choice of therapy depends on the severity of disease at the time of diagnosis and may be adjusted depending on how patients respond to certain treatments. Clinicians caring for patients with IBD often set their own definitions based on clinical experience and how disruptive the disease is in the lives of their patients. Some treatments are most often used only during a flare-up, whereas others need to be taken continuously.

DIET

Researchers have studied the importance of diet in the treatment and prevention of IBD extensively; however, there is not a clear consensus on recommendations.[3] Many patients who have a diagnosis of IBD, especially those with CD, have lactose intolerance and gluten sensitivity related to inflammation of the bowel. Also, owing to the disruption of the microbiome of the gut due to treatments with antibiotics and other drugs, patients with IBD typically benefit from probiotics.

Pharmacotherapy

There are five main classes of medications used to treat IBD, as follows.

Aminosalicylates

Aminosalicylates (5-ASAs) are anti-inflammatory medications used in mild to moderate UC and CD. These medications target the lining of the intestines and are traditionally used as first-line pharmacotherapy when a patient is newly diagnosed.[5] 5-ASAs have a dose-dependent response and have been shown to not be as effective in the treatment of CD as in UC.[2] There are several different formulations of 5-ASA, with topical administration being the most beneficial. These topical agents are formulated to bypass upper GI activation and therefore target specific areas of the small intestines and colon with only one-third absorbed into the systemic circulation.[1,2] Patients with distal UC may benefit more from 5-ASA enemas or suppositories rather than oral therapy; however, combining oral and topical therapy may be more beneficial in the induction of remission in patients with UC with mild to moderate disease. These agents have shown to help patients maintain remission.[1]

Glucocorticoids

Glucocorticoids are anti-inflammatory medications used to treat moderate to severe flare-ups of UC and CD. These medications act by slowing down several inflammatory pathways and can be given by several different routes, including oral, subcutaneous (SC), or intravenous (IV), depending on the need of the patient.[2,5] These medications are not usually prescribed for long-term usage or maintenance therapy because of a range of reversible and irreversible side effects. Budesonide is a controlled-release glucocorticoid with high first-pass metabolism in the liver and therefore fewer systemic adverse effects. This drug can be effective in the induction of remission in mild to moderate CD and UC.[1,2]

Immunomodulators or immunosuppressants

Immunomodulators or immunosuppressants are medications that exert their effects through modification of the body's normal immune response. These medications are used to control severe symptoms or to help taper a steroid-dependent patient off glucocorticoids. Clinicians use these medications in combination with biological agents to control flare-ups and to maintain remission in patients.[2,5] Regular monitoring of complete blood cell count and liver enzymes is required of patients taking these medications owing to significant side effects, including bone marrow toxicity, leukopenia, and rarely, hepatosplenic T cell lymphoma. Azathioprine and mercaptopurine are effective in maintaining remission in patients with UC. Methotrexate may be used in patients with steroid-dependent CD to help alleviate symptoms and maintain remission. Researches note that methotrexate is not shown to be effective in UC; however, the reason is unclear.[1,2]

Biological agents

Biological agents are medications made from a living source; they are complex proteins used to bind to or block specific targets. There are 7 types of biologics approved by the US Food and Drug Administration (FDA) to treat IBD. These medications must be given orally, SC, or by IV infusion. The types of biological agents include tumor necrosis factor (TNF)-α inhibitors, which bind and block TNF-α; integrin receptor antagonists (antiadhesion agents); and interleukin (IL)-12 and IL-23 antagonists.[5] TNF-alpha inhibitors including infliximab, adalimumab, and certolizumab are used to treat CD, whereas infliximab, adalimumab, and golimumab are used in the treatment of UC. Patients can receive infliximab only by IV infusion, whereas adalimumab, certolizumab, and golimumab are given SC.[1,2] Antiadhesion agents natalizumab and vedolizumab are used in the treatment of moderate to severe CD, and vedolizumab is used in the treatment of moderate to severe UC. Ustekinumab, a monoclonal antibody that blocks the biological activity of IL-12 and IL-23, is used in the treatment of severe CD when TNF-alpha inhibitors have failed.[1] Before initiation of TNF-alpha inhibitors, patients should undergo testing for latent tuberculosis owing to the increased risk for reactivation during therapy. Patients should also be evaluated for chronic hepatitis B infection.[1,2]

Biosimilars

Biosimilars are biological therapies made from natural proteins that target the immune system; they are made to be nearly identical to the current biological agents. Biosimilars are approved by the FDA to treat both UC and CD; however, at the time of this publishing, they do not have the interchangeability designation approval, which means that a biosimilar cannot be substituted for a prescribed biological agent without first notifying the patient's health care provider.[6]

Step-Up versus Step-Down Therapy

Over the last decade there have been significant discussions on whether patients with IBD should be treated in a step-up therapy manner or if a step-down approach is more beneficial. In step-up therapy, which is also called "fail first" therapy, a patient begins with the most inexpensive medication first, and if therapy fails, they then move to the next most inexpensive medication.[7] Although step-up therapy may save money on prescription medications, it has not shown to save money overall because patients generally need to follow-up with the practitioner more often.[7]

The American Gastroenterology Association (AGA) standard of care is to treat the patient based on the severity of the disease with the best available therapy at the time of diagnosis. The AGA standard of care is based on evidence that patients often experience complications due to unchecked inflammation while taking suboptimal medications. This inflammation can cause scarring and permanent damage. The AGA believes that the choice of therapy should be left to the clinical practitioner.[7] This approach may sometimes be referred to as step-down therapy because practitioners may start with a combination of medications and slowly remove agents as the patient's disease becomes controlled.

Surgery

Surgery for UC is usually curative but involves removing the whole colon and rectum. Surgery is therefore typically reserved for patients with fulminant colitis, megacolon, pancolitis (or patients with left-sided colitis who are at risk for developing colon cancer), or those who have failed to respond to extensive conservative management. For patients with CD, there is no surgical cure because the disease is generally not limited to one area of the GI tract. Instead, surgery is mainly reserved to treat complications of CD including a fistula that cannot be healed by medication alone, a stricture causing obstruction, a refractory area of disease, or cancer. Nevertheless, approximately 66% to 75% of patients with CD will end up needing surgery at some point in their clinical course, with 50% of patients experiencing a return of their symptoms within 4 years. For this reason, it is recommended that patients with CD who undergo surgery receive aggressive therapy with TNF-alpha inhibitors and/or immunomodulators following surgery with the goal to prevent recurrence.[1,8]

Prognosis

Fortunately, fewer than 5% of patients with IBD will have a continuous course of active disease. In comparison, 13% of patients will have a relapse-free course. Poor prognostic factors for patients with UC include, but are not limited to, age less than 40 years at diagnosis, severe endoscopic disease, elevated CRP levels, low serum albumin level, and a history of ex-smoking. For patients with CD, poor prognostic factors include, but are not limited to, age less than 30 years at diagnosis, perianal/severe rectal disease, penetrating or stenosis disease, and active smoking.[8]

DISCUSSION

Chronic inflammatory diseases, autoimmune or otherwise, exhibit two cardinal features: variability (due to the intrinsic heterogeneity of the affected individuals and the surrounding environment in which they live) and complexity (due to the seemingly endless number of factors and mechanisms associated with the disease). These two features are inextricably intertwined, giving rise to inconsistencies and unpredictably in (1) how a disease clinically manifests, (2) the outcomes of chosen therapeutic interventions, and (3) how one anticipates and prevents flare-ups. For these reasons alone, one could argue that the care of all patients with IBD is complex.[9]

The care of patients with IBD requires coordination between gastroenterologists, surgeons, mental health practitioners, dieticians, and many other health care providers. The health care system is often difficult to navigate, which may give rise to psychological stress. Since the 1930s, the relationship between IBD and stress has been recognized. At this time, IBD was considered a purely psychosomatic disease. Today, the exact role of stress in the onset of IBD is not established. What has been established, however, is that stress is a triggering and exacerbating factor in relation to the course and symptoms of IBD (ie, it is one of the determinants of disease relapse).[9–11]

The unpredictable, uncertain, and chronic course of IBD can also cause psychological and interpersonal issues for patients. These include losing control of the bowel, fatigue, impairment of body image, fearing sexual inadequacy, social isolation, dependency, concern about not reaching one's full potential, and feeling dirty. Psychological disorders such as anxiety and depression are also common among patients with IBD, as are psychological side effects to most current conventional medical therapies. It is for these reasons that the health-related quality of life of patients with IBD is substantially impaired. Patients with IBD may benefit from integrating psychological treatment (including cognitive therapy and/or antidepressant medications) with conventional medical therapy, especially in the current climate. At the time of publication, the severe acute respiratory syndrome coronavirus-2 (coronavirus disease 2019) pandemic was prominent. Not only are patients with IBD actively advised on the need to shield at home during this time, the counseling of patients regarding treatment becomes a much more complex task (eg, there are significant risks associated with introducing a new immunosuppressive medication during a global pandemic).[9–11]

SPECIAL PATIENT GROUP: PREGNANT AND BREASTFEEDING

In the United States, approximately 0.5% of the population, or 1.6 million people, have IBD. Of those, roughly half are women, and most will carry the diagnosis during their reproductive years. Owing to fears about the disease and its effect on pregnancy (miscarriage, premature delivery, poor maternal weight gain, and so forth), 17% of women with IBD are voluntarily childless compared with 6% of the general population.[12–14]

Medical therapies, including biological agents and corticosteroids, do not decrease a woman's fertility. In comparison, active disease at conception (the biggest risk factor; complicates 30%–35% of all IBD pregnancies) and a history of certain surgeries (ie, proctectomy, permanent ostomies and ileal pouch-anal anastomosis [IPAA]), have both been shown to have a negative correlation. Ideally, women should be in remission for six months before conceiving. Assisted reproductive technology in women with CD or UC is also not as effective versus infertile women without IBD.[12,13]

During pregnancy, care of women with IBD should be shared between a gastroenterologist and an obstetric provider, including at least one consultation visit with a maternal fetal medicine specialist. Most medical therapy for IBD should be continued for several reasons including (1) decreasing disease activity, (2) reducing the likelihood of flare-ups, and (3) lowering the incidence of adverse pregnancy outcomes. Some known medications to avoid include rifaximin (antibiotic; teratogenicity described in animal models), methotrexate (immunomodulator; contraindicated), and tofacitinib (immunomodulator; limited human data). If on sulfasalazine, it is recommended that the pregnant female take folate supplementation due to impaired folic acid absorption and metabolism. Methotrexate and tofacitinib are also contraindicated when breastfeeding. Most other IBD medications are either undetectable or present low concentrations in breast milk such that breastfeeding is encouraged in all patients with IBD. Surgery in patients with UC during pregnancy should be performed only for emergency indications, including severe hemorrhage, perforation, and megacolon refractory to medical therapy. Total colectomy and ileostomy carry a 50% risk of postoperative spontaneous abortion, and fetal mortality is also high in patients with CD requiring surgery.[12–14]

Most patients with IBD can undergo a vaginal delivery. Patients with active perianal CD, a previous rectovaginal tear/fistula, or a history of IPAA surgery, however, should be considered for cesarean delivery. The infants of mothers with IBD should also be given all vaccines (in keeping with Centers for Disease Control and Prevention guidelines) except for the rotavirus vaccine if the mother received biological agents (except certolizumab) during the third trimester.[12,13]

SPECIAL PATIENT GROUP: CHILDREN

CD and UC are often diagnosed in adolescence and young adulthood, with a rising incidence in children (4% of patients with IBD first present before age five years and 18% before age ten years). With a prevalence of 100 to 200 per 100,000 children in the United States (estimated 70,000 total), most pediatricians will encounter children with IBD in their general practice.[15–17]

Although children can present with classical symptoms, 22% present atypically with growth failure, anemia, perianal disease, or other EM. Physical examination (which may provide clues to underlying pathologic features) must include assessment of growth curves. Some children present with acute weight loss, whereas others present with a more insidious flattening of their weight and height curves. Conversely, 25% of children with IBD are clinically obese at the time of diagnosis. On laboratory examination, common abnormal findings in children include anemia, thrombocytosis, hypoalbuminemia, and elevated inflammatory markers. However, approximately 10% to 20% of children with IBD will have normal laboratory results. Fecal calprotectin (a neutrophil-derived protein with elevated concentrations in the setting of intestinal inflammation) has emerged as a useful biomarker in children with IBD with 98% sensitivity and 68% specificity.[15–17]

When a primary care clinician suspects IBD in a child based on their clinical and/or laboratory findings, they should promptly refer that child to a pediatric gastroenterologist for endoscopic evaluation. Esophagogastroduodenoscopy and ileocolonoscopy with biopsy remain the criterion standard for diagnosis and classification. After endoscopic diagnosis, small bowel imaging should also be performed to (1) help map disease location, (2) assess disease severity, and (3) identify complications such as fistulas, abscesses, and intestinal strictures.[15,16]

The goals of treatment of children with IBD include (1) eliminating symptoms and restoring quality of life, (2) restoring normal growth, and (3) eliminating complications while minimizing the adverse effects of medications. These goals have changed dramatically in the past 20 to 25 years in line with new medication developments and large collaborative research efforts. Unique considerations when treating children with IBD include paying attention to the effects of the disease on (1) growth and development (growth failure occurs in approximately 40% and 10% of children with CD and UC, respectively), (2) bone health (abnormalities in bone metabolism and achieving optimal adult bone mass), and (3) psychosocial functioning (higher rates of depressive and anxiety disorders).[15,16]

In children, corticosteroids are effective for the induction of clinical remission in CD and UC; however, approximately half of patients will either become dependent on corticosteroids or go on to require surgery. Also, fewer than one-third of patients with CD in clinical remission with corticosteroid treatment will achieve mucosal healing. Although aminosalicylates have been used for more than 40 years as an alternative to corticosteroids for the treatment of IBD, few clinical trials have been conducted in children. The current research, however, does show that 30% of children with UC will maintain remission with administration of aminosalicylates alone. Although commonly prescribed in CD, systematic reviews do not support their efficacy. In children with UC refractory to aminosalicylates, the use of thiopurine drugs is supported. In a similar manner, the introduction of mercaptopurine has been shown to reduce corticosteroid exposure and improve the maintenance of clinical remission in children with CD. Finally, the introduction of TNF-alpha inhibitor therapy has revolutionized the treatment of IBD in children in recent years. TNF-alpha inhibitors are typically used in children with IBD refractory to corticosteroids or in those who are corticosteroid dependent despite immunomodulator therapy.[15,16]

As in adults, surgery is an important therapeutic option in the comprehensive management of UC and CD in children. Children with UC refractory to medical therapy may undergo a total colectomy with IPAA with excellent long-term outcomes. Surgery in children with CD is reserved for those with complications, and in some cases, when disease is refractory to medical therapy. Among children with CD, 14% require intra-abdominal surgery within five years of diagnosis.[15,16]

SPECIAL PATIENT GROUP: ELDERLY

Considering the aging population, the incidence and prevalence of elderly-onset IBD (defined as new onset of disease after age 60 years) is likely set to increase. Unfortunately, there is a relative lack of data specific to elderly patients with IBD due to their exclusion from most clinical trials. This lack of data can make clinical decision making somewhat challenging in this already vulnerable population as treatment paradigms are still being developed and improved. For these reasons, higher disease-related mortality has been reported in patients with elderly-onset UC and CD than in patients with early-onset disease (defined as new onset of disease before age 60 years).[18-20]

Most patients (65%) with elderly-onset IBD are diagnosed during the sixth decade of life, 25% are diagnosed during the seventh decade, and a further 10% during the eighth decade. Although the clinical features and natural history of the disease at these ages is like those of younger patients, there are some significant differences to be aware of, including a broader differential diagnosis. According to the literature, misdiagnosis may occur in up to 60% of elderly patients with IBD when compared with 15% of younger patients, with a delay in diagnosis of up to six years. A familial history of IBD is less common with elderly-onset IBD, and the prevalence of EM is also lower, varying from 0% to 7%.[19,20]

Treatment of elderly patients with IBD is complex. Age-specific concerns, such as comorbidities, polypharmacy, and worsening locomotor and cognitive function must be considered. For unknown reasons, the most used medications in elderly patients with IBD are aminosalicylates, which are prescribed in 60% to 90% of patients with UC and 30% to 90% of patients with CD, respectively. The combination of oral and topical aminosalicylates is more effective than oral therapy alone; however, age-related physical limitations may affect an older patient's ability to use topical therapy correctly. Steroid therapy is used in up to one-third of elderly patients with IBD, and overall rates of immunomodulator and biological agents use are lower in elderly patients with UC and CD than in patients with early-onset disease. According to international consensus guidelines, any patient on, or very likely to commence, meaningful immunosuppressive therapy for control of their IBD should be routinely vaccinated. In general, elderly patients are at an increased risk of infection due to a myriad of reasons.[19,20]

Surgery plays an important role in the overall management of patients with elderly-onset IBD, especially in those who have failed medical therapy. Careful patient selection and optimal timing is key to ensuring the best possible outcomes. In patients with elderly-onset UC, surgical rates are higher than in those with early-onset UC. Total colectomy with permanent ileostomy is the most performed procedure. Total colectomy with IPAA is the surgical procedure of choice in elderly-onset UC, but only in patients who have good anal sphincter function with no history of fecal incontinence. For CD, overall surgery rates are similar in early-onset and elderly-onset patients.[19,20]

ORIGINAL CASE STUDY

Mr X is a 28-year-old white male with CD. His story began when he was as a sophomore in high school. He was outside walking to class one day when his right eye swelled and shut abruptly. He was immediately taken by his parents to an ophthalmologist where he was diagnosed with conjunctivitis and given antibiotic eye drops. A few weeks later, Mr X developed flulike symptoms and started to lose an unspecified amount of weight. Over the course of the next year he visited multiple specialists where multiple tests were run, all coming back inconclusive. Mr X then developed mouth ulcers and bloody diarrhea with no prior history. He was eventually referred to gastroenterology for a colonoscopy, which showed no colonic changes.

Six months later, Mr X developed sacroiliac pain and was referred to rheumatology. The rheumatology physician assistant (PA) ordered an MRI scan, which revealed ankylosing spondylitis. The PA also suggested a repeat colonoscopy, which revealed the diagnosis of CD. Mr X was immediately administered infliximab, which took 3 hours to administer via infusion. Infliximab controlled Mr X's symptoms, and he started to regain weight. Mr X remained on infliximab for one year until he was switched to certolizumab. The rationale for changing his treatment regimen was that Mr X was shortly leaving home for college. Mr X was taught how to inject himself and has been compliant with this medication ever since. In terms of daily living, Mr X no longer eats red meat or gluten because he has found that these foods cause his CD to flare-up. Mr X is otherwise doing well.

SUMMARY

The management of all patients with IBD, whether they have CD or UC, is complex. Understanding of IBD, in addition to choices and goals of available therapy, are constantly evolving. Special patient groups, namely, children, the elderly, and women who are pregnant or breastfeeding, present a unique challenge. These patients must be cared for in a timely and effective manner to prevent (1) psychological stress, (2) a worsening in clinical condition, and (3) the need for more comprehensive medical treatment or surgical intervention.

CLINICS CARE POINTS

- In pregnant women, most medical therapy for IBD can be continued.
- Most IBD medications are either undetectable or present low concentrations in breast milk such that breastfeeding is encouraged in all patients with IBD.
- Most patients with IBD who are pregnant can undergo a vaginal delivery without complication.
- There is a rising incidence of IBD in children, with 22% of patients presenting atypically.
- Endoscopic evaluation followed by small bowel imaging remain the criterion standard for the diagnosis and classification of IBD in children.
- For children with IBD, the goals of treatment are to (1) eliminate symptoms and restore quality of life, (2) restore normal growth, and (3) eliminate complications while minimizing the adverse effects of medications.
- Misdiagnosis may occur in up to 60% of elderly patients with IBD when compared with 15% of younger patients, giving rise to higher disease-related mortality.
- Treatment of elderly patients with IBD is complex, especially given age-specific concerns, such as comorbidities, polypharmacy, and worsening locomotor and cognitive function.
- Surgery plays an important role in the overall management of patients with elderly-onset IBD, especially in those who have failed medical therapy.

DISCLOSURE

The authors have nothing to disclose.

REFERENCES

1. MKSAP18: medical Knowledge Self-assessment Program; Gastroenterology and Hepatology. In: Masters P, editor. 18th edition. Philadelphia: American College of Physicians; 2018.
2. Ananthakrishnan AN, Xavier RJ, Podolsky DK. Inflammatory bowel diseases: a clinician's guide. John Wiley & Sons, Incorporated; 2017. Available at: http://ebookcentral.proquest.com/lib/lmunet/detail.action?docID=4818683. Accessed October 16, 2020.

3. Levine A, Rhodes JM, Lindsay JO, et al. Dietary guidance for patients with inflammatory bowel disease from the international organization for the study of inflammatory bowel disease. Clin Gastroenterol Hepatol 2020;18(6):1381–92.

4. Nemati S, Teimourian S. An overview of inflammatory bowel disease: general consideration and genetic screening approach in diagnosis of early onset subsets. Middle East J Dig Dis 2017;9(2):69–80.

5. What patients need to know about living with IBD. Clin Gastroenterol Hepatol 2020;18(2):A15.

6. Biosimilars. Clin Gastroenterol Hepatol 2020;18(1):A34.

7. Michael L, Weinstein MD. Put Patients First by Reforming Step therapy Protocols. Gastroenterology & Endoscopy News. Available at: https://www.gastro endonews.com/Opinions-and-Letters/Article/05-18/Reforming-Step-Therapy-Protocols/48628.

8. O'Connell CB, Cogan-Drew T, editors. A comprehensive review for the certification and recertification examinations for physician assistants. 6th edition. Philadelphia: Wolters Kluwer; 2018.

9. Fiocchi C. Inflammatory bowel disease: complexity and variability need integration. Front Med 2018;5:75.

10. Sajadinejad MS, Asgari K, Molavi H, et al. Psychological issues in inflammatory bowel disease: an overview. Gastroenterol Res Pract 2012;2012:1–11.

11. Christian K, Cross RK. Improving outcomes in patients with inflammatory bowel disease through integrated multi-disciplinary care—the future of IBD care. Clin Gastroenterol Hepatol 2018;16(11):1708–9.

12. Veerisetty SS, Eschete SO, Uhlhorn A-P, et al. Women's Health in Inflammatory Bowel Disease. Am J Med Sci 2018;356(3):227–33.

13. De Felice KM, Kane SV. Inflammatory bowel disease in women of reproductive age. Expert Rev Gastroenterol Hepatol 2014;8(4):417–25.

14. Mahadevan U, Robinson C, Bernasko N, et al. Inflammatory bowel disease in pregnancy clinical care pathway: a report from the American gastroenterological association IBD parenthood project working group. Gastroenterology 2019;156(5):1508–24.

15. Rosen MJ, Dhawan A, Saeed SA. Inflammatory bowel disease in children and adolescents. JAMA Pediatr 2015;169(11):1053.

16. Oliveira SB, Monteiro IM. Diagnosis and management of inflammatory bowel disease in children. BMJ 2017;357:j2083.

17. Moazzami B, Moazzami K, Rezaei N. Early onset inflammatory bowel disease: manifestations, genetics and diagnosis. TurkJPediatr 2019;61(5):637.

18. Olén O, Askling J, Sachs MC, et al. Mortality in adult-onset and elderly-onset IBD: a nationwide register-based cohort study 1964–2014. Gut 2020;69(3):453–61.

19. Kedia S, Limdi JK, Ahuja V. Management of inflammatory bowel disease in older persons: evolving paradigms. Intest Res 2018;16(2):194.

20. LeBlanc J-F, Wiseman D, Lakatos PL, et al. Elderly patients with inflammatory bowel disease: updated review of the therapeutic landscape. World J Gastroenterol 2019;25(30):4158–71.

Nonalcoholic Fatty Liver Disease: The New Epidemic

Michael Bessette, MD

KEYWORDS

- Cirrhosis • Fatty liver • MAFLD • NAFLD • NASH • Nonalcoholic fatty liver disease
- Nonalcoholic steatohepatitis • Steatosis

KEY POINTS

- Nonalcoholic fatty liver disease (NAFLD) is a chronic liver disease caused by triglyceride accumulation triggered by obesity and insulin resistance.
- NALFD will soon become the leading cause of liver failure worldwide.
- Treatment is based on weight reduction through diet and exercise, or bariatric surgery.

INTRODUCTION

Nonalcoholic fatty liver disease (NAFLD) is a spectrum of disorders related to triglyceride infiltration of hepatocytes not owing to other causes, such as alcohol use, other toxic medications or substances, viral hepatitis, or starvation. Alcohol use is defined as more than 1 drink (10 g of ethanol) per day for women and 2 drinks per day for men.[1] The presence of excess triglycerides in the hepatocytes is the most benign version but can result in cirrhosis in the most malignant cases.

DISCUSSION
Epidemiology

NAFLD is the fastest growing cause of liver failure in the world. It is currently one of the top 3 pathologic conditions requiring liver transplantation, along with alcoholic cirrhosis and viral hepatitis. The rate of increase will make it the primary reason for liver failure in the United States within the next 5 years. Current estimates from imaging studies place the prevalence of NAFLD at 25% in the US population.[2] Racial variations show a lower incidence in black Americans and a higher incidence in Hispanic Americans as compared with white, non-Hispanic Americans.[2] The presence of obesity, insulin resistance, or metabolic syndrome increases the risk of development of NAFLD by up to 2.3-fold.[2]

Physician Assistant Program, Bouvé College, Northeastern University, 202 Robinson Hall, 360 Huntington Avenue, Boston, MA 02115, USA
E-mail address: m.bessette@northeastern.edu

Physician Assist Clin 6 (2021) 667–675
https://doi.org/10.1016/j.cpha.2021.05.010
2405-7991/21/© 2021 Elsevier Inc. All rights reserved.

Cirrhosis is unlikely in those with only signs of fatty infiltration. However, as inflammation, hepatocellular death, and fibrosis progress, as in nonalcoholic steatohepatitis (NASH), the risk of cirrhosis and primary liver cancer increases. In those with cirrhosis, the risk of primary cancer is 3% annually.[3] NASH can have variable progression and even regression before cirrhotic tissue damage develops. However, primary cancers have been documented in NAFLD patients who do not show signs of cirrhosis.[3]

Obesity and insulin resistance are risk factors for NAFLD at any age. The disease, in all its forms, has been documented in children, adolescents, adults, and the elderly. The mechanism of progression is not well understood. For this reason, prevention and treatment are focused on risk factor control. Slowing the progression of liver disease will largely rely on gains in the fight against childhood obesity.

Genetic factors may be responsible for up to half of the risk of developing fatty liver and the subsequent inflammatory damage according to twin studies. Several genes have been identified as culprits. PNPLA3 encodes for an enzyme that moves lipids between cells. It is found more often in those with fatty liver, cirrhosis, and primary liver cancer.[2] Other gene-related lipid homeostases are also being studied as possible causes for the development of NAFLD.[2]

Worldwide Incidence

Obesity is accelerating across the planet. There are more than 1 billion overweight adults and more than 300 million cases of obesity.[4] NAFLD is the most common liver disease in Western countries and is the fastest growing chronic liver disease worldwide.[4] The global cost of care will continue to increase. The fastest growing segment is in obese children.[4] Industrialized areas show increased rates possibly because of the added effects of environmental toxins. Genetic factors place Hispanics and Native Americans at even higher risk. Global efforts to control obesity and manage metabolic syndromes will be the keys to control the epidemic rise of NAFLD.[1]

Pathologic Condition

The basis of NAFLD is triglyceride deposition in hepatocytes. In its simplest form, the synthesis of triglycerides in the hepatocytes is greater than the degradation. There are several factors that can lead to the imbalance in handling of triglycerides by the liver. Obesity triggers accumulation of triglycerides. The mechanism is circular and progressive. Obesity is paired with increased calorie uptake through increased intestinal permeability and changes in the gut microbiome. The alteration in the gut barrier exposes the liver to more intestinal content by-products. The liver responds by producing inflammatory proteins that decrease insulin uptake by cells. Adipose deposits also produce adipokines that increase insulin resistance. The insulin resistance causes hyperglycemia. The hyperglycemia triggers the pancreas to produce more insulin. The increased insulin triggers more triglyceride production and storage, and the liver gets more and more fatty (**Fig. 1**).

It must then be considered how the accumulation of triglycerides causes the inflammation characteristic of NASH and the fibrous damage of cirrhosis. Triglycerides alone are not toxic to hepatocytes. However, the fatty acid precursors and the oxygen, free-radical metabolites can cause hepatocyte damage (lipotoxicity), Hormonal mediators and inflammatory cytokines are stimulated by lipotoxicity. Hepatocyte regeneration is inhibited by these proteins, resulting in cell death. The dying cells release more toxic proteins that inhibit the growth of new liver cells. Myofibroblasts and progenitor cells are produced and begin to remodel the damaged liver area with either new hepatocytes or fibrous cells. The variability of the regeneration process creates the mottled histology found in NASH. If the process creates excess of fibrous tissue, cirrhosis

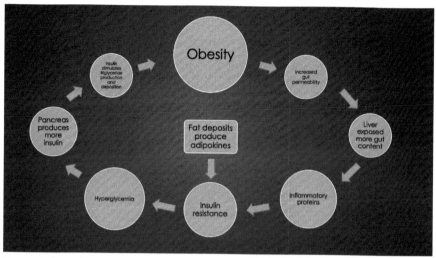

Fig. 1. Triglyceride and fatty liver cycle.

ensues. Increased rates of cell damage and regeneration foster a favorable environment for deregulation of cell growth resulting in primary liver cancers. Medical professionals and researchers have not yet found what determines if a hepatocyte will regenerate as a normal cell, a fibrous scar, or a malignant cell. The obscurity of the process limits testing and treatment development. Therefore, prevention of triglyceride buildup is the basis of current clinical care.

Evaluation

Fatty liver is diagnosed by demonstrating fat accumulation in hepatocytes. Because it is most often asymptomatic, the diagnosis is typically an incidental finding while imaging for other concerns. However, an increased level of attention to the risk factors can prompt a good provider to screen for fatty liver in the appropriate patient population. The Fatty Liver Index (FLI) was developed to aid in patient screening[5] (**Fig. 2**). All patients with repeated elevated liver enzymes, obesity, or insulin resistance should have an FLI performed and further testing influenced by the score. Imaging should be performed on those with an intermediate or high FLI.[2]

Ultrasound is a cost-effective, first-line screening option. Computed tomography (CT) and MRI are both more accurate and more expensive. Diagnosis of NAFLD in the patient with fatty liver on imaging requires exclusion of other causes of fat infiltration. Alcohol consumption must be less than 1 drink per day for women and 2 drinks per day for men. A drink is defined as 10 g of ethanol as is typical in 12 ounces of beer, 4 ounces of wine, or 1.5 ounces of distilled spirits. **Box 1** shows a listing of common drugs that can cause fatty liver. Other causes of liver disease must be excluded, such as viral hepatitis, autoimmune hepatitis, alpha 1 antitrypsin deficiency, Wilson disease, and hemochromatosis. Liver size and hepatic transaminases may be normal in patients with NAFLD.

Staging disease severity in NAFLD patients is critically important. Those with simple steatosis will do well with conservative management. However, it is vital to recognize those who show signs of liver inflammation and scarring consistent with NASH, as they will need more aggressive management and monitoring. A history of risk factors for metabolic disease and physical findings of liver dysfunction including the stigmata

Fatty Liver Index (FLI) = e^x / (1 + e^y) × 100
Where y = 0.953 × ln(triglycerides, mg/dL) + 0.139 × BMI, kg/m^2 + 0.718 × ln (GGT, U/L) + 0.053 × waist circumference, cm – 15.745

Fatty Liver Index	Risk	Diagnosis
<30	Low	Fatty liver ruled out (LR- = 0.2)
30 to <60	Indeterminate	Fatty liver neither ruled in nor ruled out
≥60	High	Fatty liver ruled in (LR+ = 4.3)

Fig. 2. FLI.

of portal hypertension and hormone deficiencies will lead the clinician to suspect liver fibrosis. Fibrosis is scored from 0 to 4 based on the METAVIR scoring system (F0, no fibrosis; F1, portal fibrosis; F2, periportal fibrosis; F3, bridging fibrosis; F4, cirrhosis).[6] Although liver biopsy remains the gold standard for staging of fibrosis, there are now less-invasive measures that can be used to determine which patients require advanced imaging and possible biopsy.[3] The NAFLD-Fibrosis score[7] (**Fig. 3**) and the Fibrosis-4 (FIB-4) score[6] (**Fig. 4**) have been shown to be equally effective in screening for high-risk patients.[5,8] Patients with fibrosis scores of less than 1.455 are low risk and may continue with regular follow-up. Those with scores greater than 1.455 should be sent for advanced studies to determine the level of fibrosis.[8] Elastography is recommended to further stage intermediate- and high-risk individuals.[8] Vibration-controlled transient elastography is the most widely used and best validated study. Magnetic resonance elastography shows the most promise for high sensitivity and ability to delineate the anatomy, but it is costly and will cause problems for claustrophobic patients. Those patients with signs of intermediate to advanced fibrosis on elastography should have liver biopsy for confirmation and staging. Patients with nondiagnostic elastography studies should also go for liver biopsy for proper staging.[3]

Thorough evaluation of NAFLD patients should include considerations of screening for hepatocellular carcinoma (HCC). The incidence of HCC in NAFLD patients without cirrhosis is much lower than those with cirrhosis (0.08/1000 person-years vs 10.6/1000 person-years).[3] HCC screening is recommended in those with fibrosis stage 3 or 4. Ultrasound screening should be done every 6 months. Alpha-fetoprotein testing has not been shown to improve the sensitivity of HCC screening over imaging alone in patients with NAFLD.[9] Obesity, tobacco, and alcohol use will all increase the risk of developing HCC in NAFLD patients, and efforts should be encouraged to remediate those risks.[8]

Therapeutic Options

Management of NAFLD and NASH currently focuses on reducing the triggers of inflammation. Obesity is the primary cause of the cascade leading to fatty liver. Weight

Box 1
Medications and toxins that can cause hepatic steatosis

Anti-infectious agents
- Doxycycline
- HAART
- Tetracycline

Cardiac compounds
- Amiodarone
- Hydralazine
- Perhexiline maleate

Cytotoxic and cytostatic compounds
- L-Asparaginase
- Azacitidine
- Azaserine
- Bleomycin
- Methotrexate
- Puromycin

Hormonals and steroids
- 4,4'-Diethylaminoethoxyhexesterol
- Ethionine
- Estrogens
- Glucocorticoids
- Tamoxifen

Metals
- Antimony
- Barium salts
- Chromates
- Ethyl bromide
- Phosphorus
- Rare earth metals
- Thallium compounds
- Uranium compounds

Other toxins
- Hypoglycin (unripe fruit of the Ackee tree)
- Orotate
- Safrole (found in Ecstasy and herbal supplements)

▶ **Requires: AST, ALT, Platelet count, Albumin**

▶ **Formula :**

▶ $-1.675 + 0.037 \times$ age (years) $+ 0.094 \times$ BMI (kg/m2) $+ 1.13 \times$ IFG/diabetes (yes = 1, no = 0) $+ 0.99 \times$ AST/ALT ratio $- 0.013 \times$ platelet ($\times 109$/l) $- 0.66 \times$ albumin (g/dl)

▶ **Explanation of Result :**

▶ NAFLD Score $< -1.455 =$ F0-F2
NAFLD Score $-1.455 - 0.675 =$ indeterminate score
NAFLD Score $> 0.675 =$ F3-F4

Fig. 3. NAFLD fibrosis score.

- FIB-4 Score = (Age* x AST) / (Platelets x √(ALT))
- *Use with caution in patients <35 or >65 y old, as the score has been shown to be less reliable in these patients.

FIB-4 Score	Approximate fibrosis stage*
<1.45	0–1
1.45–3.25	2–3
>3.25	4

Fig. 4. FIB-4 score.

reduction has been recommended despite lack of consistent evidence. A weight reduction of at least 5% is advised for most patients. Better evidence supports a Mediterranean diet that is low in sugar and processed carbohydrates. Increased omega-3 intake has been shown to decrease insulin resistance and reduce triglyceride accumulation in the liver. Coffee is beneficial as an antioxidant, and 2 to 3 cups per day are recommended.[8] Alcohol avoidance will decrease the risk of developing HCC, although studies have shown that mild alcohol use may be beneficial in reducing the development of fibrosis in NASH patients.[8]

Exercise is a first-line recommendation in NAFLD patients. Studies have shown benefits that are independent of diet changes. These benefits include reduction of hepatic triglycerides, transaminases, and insulin resistance. Both aerobic and resistance-based exercises were equally effective.[10] An exercise program should include 150 to 200 minutes of activity per week. The activity may be any combination of aerobic and resistance formats.[11]

Bariatric surgery has proven to be an effective treatment for obesity. The positive effects carry over to NAFLD and NASH. Studies have shown beneficial effects on steatosis, inflammation, and fibrosis in most patients after bariatric surgery. The effects are progressive and have been documented out to 5 years after surgery.[12] However, the data are retrospective and of low quality; therefore, further studies are needed to confirm the benefits. If bariatric surgery is considered, it should be done before there is significant cirrhosis. Cirrhosis increases the complication rates significantly and may exclude the patient from qualifying for bariatric surgery.[12]

Lipid-lowering agents have shown mixed results in clinical trials. Statins, although effective at lowering serum triglyceride levels, have not shown any benefit in reducing hepatic triglycerides, reducing inflammation, or improving fibrosis.[13] Statins are safe for use in patients with NASH, diabetes, and even mildly elevated transaminases and should be considered for treatment of high cholesterol.[14] Omega-3 supplements may show some benefit in reducing fatty liver, but the current data are inadequate.[14]

Metformin is currently the most prescribed medication for insulin resistance. It is effective for lowering hyperglycemia, cholesterol levels, and transaminases, but it has not been effective in improving steatosis or fibrosis, and inflammation may increase.[14] Pioglitazone has been the subject of several trials for treatment of NAFLD. Meta-analysis of the data showed reduction of hepatic steatosis, inflammation, hepatocellular ballooning, and modest improvement in fibrosis in both diabetic and nondiabetic patients.[14] There are some safety concerns regarding weight gain, osteoporosis, and increased risk of bladder cancer.[15]

Vitamin E and vitamin C have been studied to explore if the anti-inflammatory properties would be beneficial in NASH patients. Vitamin E alone is beneficial in nondiabetic adult patients in reducing steatosis and inflammation.[16] In nondiabetic children, it reduced hepatocellular ballooning but did not improve steatosis or inflammation.[16] Vitamin C alone has not shown consistent improvement in any markers of NASH pathologic condition. However, there is good evidence that vitamin C deficiency significantly increases the risk of developing NAFLD.[16] The findings are more pronounced in men and nonobese patients.[16] The combination of vitamins E and C showed improvement in inflammation and fibrosis in adults and children.[16] Combined with atorvastatin, there was a 71% reduction in the development of NASH in those with NAFLD.[17] Studies on the long-term safety of vitamin E therapy show an increase in all-cause mortality, risk of prostate cancer, and cerebral hemorrhage.[18]

Liver transplantation is the most extreme treatment and may be the only option for patients with advanced cirrhosis from NALFD. The comorbidities often found with NAFLD, such as obesity, diabetes mellitus, and vascular disease, can limit the appropriateness of a major surgical procedure. Those who do complete liver transplant have done well. However, if the risk factors for NAFLD are not controlled after surgery, the disease may recur in the new liver.[8]

Future Directions

There is a recent push to modify NAFLD to metabolic dysfunction–associated fatty liver disease (MAFLD).[19] The goal is to better accentuate the true cause of the disease and to be more inclusive of other concomitant diseases. MAFLD can exist with other causes of liver disease, including alcohol abuse. The outcome should be a better research focus on the causes of inflammation and fibrosis and improved treatments.[19]

There are currently more than 70 trials underway for new treatments for NAFLD and NASH.[20] There are several molecules that are showing early benefit. Obeticholic acid targets intracellular bile acid receptors to better regulate the production of lipids. Phase 2b data show significant improvement in inflammation and fibrosis in NASH patients.[21] Resmetirom is a selective beta-agonist for the thyroid hormone receptor. It also showed a decrease in liver fat and improvement in NASH findings in phase 2b trials.[22] Aramchol is a bile acid conjugate that can inhibit fatty acid metabolism.[23] It has decreased liver fat and slowed the progression of NASH fibrosis in its phase 2b trials. These promising early results give hope that better treatment options will soon be available.

SUMMARY

NAFLD is rapidly becoming the number one cause of chronic liver disease and cirrhosis. Obesity and insulin resistance are the primary underlying causes. Triglyceride deposition in the liver without other causes, including excess alcohol intake, is diagnostic. All individuals with risk factors should be screened using the FLI. Those with intermediate to high scores should have imaging (ultrasound or CT) to confirm the presence of hepatic steatosis. In those with fatty liver, the metabolites and precursors of triglycerides can cause inflammation that may lead to fibrosis or development of primary liver cancer. NALFD patients should be examined for physical signs of liver inflammation and dysfunction that would indicate NASH. They can be screened for fibrosis using the FIB-4 and NAFLD-Fibrosis scoring indices and referred for elastographic imaging or biopsy if they are of intermediate or high risk, respectively. Initial treatment of NAFLD must include a diet low in sugar and refined carbohydrates, increased antioxidants such as coffee and vitamins E and C, and regular exercise of any type. Pioglitazone may be of benefit. Metformin and statins will not improve NAFLD but are useful in managing the underlying comorbid conditions and may (in the case of atorvastatin) reduce the likelihood of progressing from NAFLD to NASH.

Bariatric surgery is a useful option in those with uncontrolled obesity and NAFLD. Liver transplant is the only option for patients with severe cirrhosis owing to NASH. Transplant patients will do well and have a low recurrence of disease if the risk factors of obesity and insulin resistance are well managed.

CLINICS CARE POINTS

- Use the Fatty Liver Index to screen all patients with repeated elevated liver enzymes, obesity, and/or insulin resistance.
- Diet and exercise are the first-line treatments for nonalcoholic fatty liver disease.
- FIB-4 and Nonalcoholic Fatty Liver Disease-Fibrosis scores should be calculated on all nonalcoholic fatty liver disease patients.
- Fibrosis testing should be performed on all with intermediate or high index scores.
- Pioglitazone should be considered in patients with early nonalcoholic steatohepatitis.
- Liver biopsy should be performed on those with high fibrosis scores or indeterminate imaging.
- Hepatocellular carcinoma screening should be done regularly in patients with moderate to severe fibrosis.
- Bariatric surgery is effective for reducing obesity and nonalcoholic fatty liver disease in patients who qualify.
- Liver transplants owing to cirrhosis from nonalcoholic steatohepatitis have low rates of recurrence if obesity and metabolic syndrome are well managed.

DISCLOSURE

Nothing to disclose.

REFERENCES

1. Chalasani N, Younossi Z, Lavine JE, et al. The diagnosis and management of non-alcoholic fatty liver disease: practice guideline by the American Association for the Study of Liver Diseases, American College of Gastroenterology, and the American Gastroenterological Association. Hepatology 2012;55(6):2005–23.
2. Younossi ZM, Koenig AB, Abdelatif D, et al. Global epidemiology of nonalcoholic fatty liver disease-meta-analytic assessment of prevalence, incidence, and outcomes. Hepatology 2016;64:73–84.
3. Kanwal F, Kramer JR, Mapakshi S, et al. Risk of hepatocellular cancer in patients with non-alcoholic fatty liver disease. Gastroenterology 2018;155(6):1828–37.e2. https://doi.org/10.1053/j.gastro.2018.08.024.
4. Arroyo-Johnson C, Mincey KD. Obesity epidemiology worldwide. Gastroenterol Clin North Am 2016;45(4):571–9. https://doi.org/10.1016/j.gtc.2016.07.012.
5. Bedogni G, Bellentani S, Miglioli L, et al. The Fatty Liver Index: a simple and accurate predictor of hepatic steatosis in the general population. BMC Gastroenterol 2006;6:33.
6. Sterling RK, Lissen E, Clumeck N, et al. Development of a simple noninvasive index to predict significant fibrosis in patients with HIV/HCV coinfection. Hepatology 2006;43:1317–25.
7. Angulo P1, Hui JM, Marchesini G, et al. The NAFLD fibrosis score: a noninvasive system that identifies liver fibrosis in patients with NAFLD. Hepatology 2007; 45(4):846–54.

8. Arab JP, Dirchwolf M, Álvares-da-Silva MR, et al. Latin American Association for the Study of the Liver (ALEH) practice guidance for the diagnosis and treatment of non-alcoholic fatty liver disease. Ann Hepatol 2020. https://doi.org/10.1016/j. aohep.2020.09.006. S1665-2681(20)30177-0.
9. Aghoram R, Cai P, Dickinson JA. Alpha-foetoprotein and/or liver ultrasonography for screening of hepatocellular carcinoma in patients with chronic hepatitis B. Cochrane Database Syst Rev 2012;(9):CD002799.
10. Orci LA, Gariani K, Oldani G, et al. Exercise-based Interventions for nonalcoholic fatty liver disease: a meta-analysis and meta-regression. Clin Gastroenterol Hepatol 2016;14(10):1398–411.
11. Orci LA, Gariani K, Oldani G, et al. Exercise-based interventions for nonalcoholic fatty liver disease: a meta-analysis and meta-regression. Clin Gastroenterol Hepatol 2016;14:1398–411.
12. Mummadi RR, Kasturi KS, Chennareddygari S, et al. Effect of bariatric surgery on nonalcoholic fatty liver disease: systematic review and meta-analysis. Clin Gastroenterol Hepatol 2008;6:1396–402.
13. Doumas M, Imprialos K, Dimakopoulou A, et al. The role of statins in the management of nonalcoholic fatty liver disease. Curr Pharm Des 2018;24(38):4587–92. https://doi.org/10.2174/1381612825666190117114305.
14. Said AA. Meta-analysis of randomized controlled trials of pharmacologic agents in non-alcoholic steatohepatitis. Ann Hepatol 2017;16:538–47.
15. Mahady SE, Webster AC, Walker S, et al. The role of thiazolidinediones in non-alcoholic steatohepatitis–a systematic review and meta-analysis. J Hepatol 2011;55:1383–90.
16. Harrison SA, Torgerson S, Hayashi P, et al. Vitamin E and vitamin C treatment improves fibrosis in patients with nonalcoholic steatohepatitis. Am J Gastroenterol 2003;98:2485–90.
17. Foster T, Budoff MJ, Saab S, et al. Atorvastatin and antioxidants for the treatment of nonalcoholic fatty liver disease: the St Francis Heart Study randomized clinical trial. Am J Gastroenterol 2011;106:71–7.
18. Sanyal AJ, Chalasani N, Kowdley KV, et al. Pioglitazone, vitamin E, or placebo for nonalcoholic steatohepatitis. N Engl J Med 2010;362:1675–85.
19. Eslam M, Sanyal AJ, George J. International Consensus Panel MAFLD: a consensus-driven proposed nomenclature for metabolic associated fatty liver disease. Gastroenterology 2020;158:1999–2014.e1.
20. [SEARCH: NAFLD]. Available at: www.clinicaltrials.gov. Accessed October 21, 2020.
21. The Farnesoid X Receptor (FXR) ligand obeticholic acid in NASH Treatment Trial(-FLINT) (FLINT) 2018 (ClinicalTrials.gov Identifier: NCT01265498). Available at: https://www.clinicaltrials.gov/ct2/show/NCT01265498?term=Obeticholic&cond=NAFLD&draw=2&rank=2. Accessed October 21, 2020.
22. A phase 3 study to evaluate the safety and biomarkers of Resmetirom (MGL-3196) in non alcoholic fatty liver disease (NAFLD) patients (MAESTRO-NAFLD1) ClinicalTrials.gov Identifier: NCT04197479. Available at: https://www.clinicaltrials.gov/ct2/show/NCT04197479?term=Resmetirom&cond=NAFLD&draw=2&rank=1. Accessed October 21, 2020.
23. Study of Aramchol in patients with fatty liver disease or nonalcoholic steatohepatitis (Aramchol003) ClinicalTrials.gov Identifier: NCT01094158. Available at: https://www.clinicaltrials.gov/ct2/show/NCT01094158?term=Aramchol&cond=NAFLD&draw=2&rank=2. Accessed October 21, 2020.

Acute Gastrointestinal Bleeding – Locating the Source and Correcting the Disorder

Matthew J. McDonald, MS, PA-C

KEYWORDS

- Upper gastrointestinal bleeding • Small bowel bleeding
- Lower gastrointestinal bleeding • Endoscopy • Colonoscopy • Hematemesis
- Melena • Hematochezia

KEY POINTS

- Gastrointestinal (GI) bleeding is categorized as either an upper GI, small bowel, or a lower GI bleeding source.
- Signs and symptoms of acute GI bleed include hematemesis, melena, hematochezia, chest pain, abdominal pain, hypotension, tachycardia, dyspnea, and syncope.
- Risk stratification scores can be helpful in determining patients who are high risk with acute upper GI bleeding, but risk stratification scores are unproven in lower GI bleeding.
- Endoscopic treatment options for acute GI bleeding include injection with saline or epinephrine, cauterization with thermal hemostatic devices, and mechanical therapy with a hemoclip or band ligation.

INTRODUCTION

Gastrointestinal (GI) bleeding is a common presenting complaint for patients in emergency and outpatient settings. In the United States, mortality associated with GI bleeding decreased from 3.78% to 2.70% between 2001 and 2009. Despite the decrease in mortality, GI bleeding continues to be a common and potentially life-threatening health issue. This article will serve as a review of current management and practice guidelines on the approach to treating nonvariceal acute upper GI bleeding, small bowel bleeding, and acute lower GI bleeding.

GI bleeding is categorized as an upper GI, small bowel, or a lower GI bleeding source. Previously, lower GI bleeding encompassed colonic and small bowel bleeding, but small bowel bleeding is being recognized as its own entity separate

School of Physician Assistant Studies, Massachusetts College of Pharmacy and Health Sciences University, Boston 179 Longwood Avenue, Griffin #423, Boston, MA 02115, USA
E-mail addresses: Matthew.mcdonald@mcphs.edu; mattmcdonaldpac@gmail.com
Twitter: @mcmattster (M.J.M.)

Physician Assist Clin 6 (2021) 677–689
https://doi.org/10.1016/j.cpha.2021.05.011
2405-7991/21/© 2021 Elsevier Inc. All rights reserved.

physicianassistant.theclinics.com

from lower GI bleeding.[2] Lower GI bleeding is now defined as bleeding from a lesion that is distal to the ileocecal valve.[2]

It is important to accurately note the clinical features of GI bleeding that suggest an overt or occult GI bleeding event. Clinical manifestations of overt GI bleeding can include hematemesis, bright red blood per rectum (hematochezia) or melena, all of which may result in hemodynamic compromise. Occult GI bleeding is described as bleeding from a GI source without any visible blood loss appreciated by the patient or health care provider. Occult GI blood loss is usually identified on fecal occult blood testing. Chronic GI bleeding and anorectal bleeding and associated disorders are beyond the scope of this publication.

Upper Gastrointestinal Bleeding

The current definition of upper GI bleeding is bleeding in the digestive tract that originates proximal to the ligament of Treitz.[4] Signs and symptoms of an upper GI bleed include hematemesis, melena, epigastric/substernal chest discomfort, acid reflux, and dysphagia. However, some patients present without any of the previously mentioned symptoms, but report fatigue, weakness, dyspnea, and lightheadedness.

The most common causes of upper GI bleeding are listed in **Table 1**. Peptic ulcer disease is the cause in approximately 50% of cases of upper GI bleeding.[5,6]

Small Bowel Bleeding

Small bowel bleeding is defined as a bleeding source distal to the ligament of Treitz, or ampulla of Vater according to some researchers, but proximal to the ileocecal valve.[7] Small bowel bleeding was previously referred to as "obscure gastrointestinal bleeding" (OGIB), and was categorized as persistent GI bleeding of unknown origin despite endoscopic evaluations of both the upper and lower GI tract.[8] Small bowel bleeding accounts for approximately 5% to 10% of all GI bleeding cases.[9] Presenting symptoms and signs can range from being overt, with melena and/or hematochezia, or occult, as evidenced by iron deficiency or heme-positive stools on guaiac testing.[10]

Patients with acute small bowel bleeding usually require more diagnostic procedures, blood transfusions, and have a much higher mortality rate than patients with upper and lower gastrointestinal bleeding.[11]

A list of common and rare etiologies of small bowel bleeding can be seen in **Table 2**.[7]

Lower GI bleeding is defined as any bleeding originating in the colon or rectum.[12] The typical signs and symptoms of a lower gastrointestinal bleed include fecal

Table 1
Etiologies of nonvariceal upper gastrointestinal bleeding

Etiology	Frequency
Peptic ulcer	26%–59%
Mallory-Weiss tear	7%–12%
Erosive gastritis/duodenitis	7%–28%
Esophagitis	4%–12%
Malignancy	4%–6%
Angiodysplasia	2%–8%
Other	2%–11%

From Samuel R, Bilal M, Tayyem O, Guturu P. Evaluation and Management of Non-Variceal Upper Gastrointestinal Bleeding. Dis Mon. 2018;64(7):333-343. https://doi.org/10.1016/j.disamonth. 2018. 02.003; With Permission.

Table 2
Common causes of small bowel bleeding

Age <40	Age >40	Rare Causes
Inflammatory bowel disease	Angioectasias	Henoch-Schoelein purpura
Dieulafoy lesions	Dieulafoy lesions	Small bowel varices/portal hypertensive enteropathy
Neoplasia	Neoplasia	Amyloidosis
Meckel diverticulum	NSAID ulcers	Blue rubber bleb nevus syndrome
Polyposis syndromes		Pseudoxanthoma elasticum
		Osler-Weber-Rendu syndrome
		Kaposi sarcoma with AIDS
		Plummer-Vinson syndrome
		Ehlers-Danlos syndrome
		Inherited polyposis syndromes
		Malignant atrophic papulosis
		Hematobilia
		Aorto-enteric fistula
		Hemosuccus entericus

From Gerson LB, Fidler JL, Cave DR, Leighton JA. ACG Clinical Guideline: Diagnosis and Management of Small Bowel Bleeding. Am J Gastroenterol. 2015;110(9):1265-1288. https://doi.org/10.1038/ajg.2015.24.

urgency, abdominal pain, hematochezia, and rarely melena (right-sided colonic sources). If the bleed is severe enough, patients may present with dyspnea, weakness, syncope, lightheadedness, hypotension, tachycardia, and signs of hypovolemia.

The most common cause of lower GI bleeding is a diverticular bleeding, accounting for approximately 50% of all cases of acute/overt lower GI bleeding.[13] Additional causes include ischemic colitis, angioectasias, malignancy, and anorectal lesions.

EPIDEMIOLOGY
Incidence/Prevalence

The incidence of upper GI bleeding seems to be declining according to current data; from 1993 to 2009, the incidence of nonvariceal upper GI bleeding decreased from 77.1 cases to 60.6 cases per 100,000 population each year.[1,14] From 2001 to 2009, there was also a decrease in lower GI bleeding from 41.8 cases to 35.7 cases per 100,000 population each year.[1]

Most studies estimate the mortality rate of upper GI bleeding to be approximately 7% to 10%,[15,16] and mortality rates in lower GI bleeding range from 2.4% to 3.9%.[17] Intensive care unit (ICU) patients who develop stress-induced ulceration resulting in upper GI bleeding have an estimated mortality rate as high as 48.5% to 65%.[18]

Risk Stratification of Gastrointestinal Bleeding

The most commonly used scores in patients who present with acute upper GI bleeding include the Glasgow Blatchford score (GBS), Clinical Rockall score, and AIMS65 score (albumin <3 g/dL, international normalized ratio [INR] >1.5, altered mental status, systolic blood pressure <90 mm Hg, and ≥65).[19] GBS uses a scoring system (0–23) based on systolic blood pressure, hemoglobin, blood urea nitrogen, melena, syncope, and the presence of heart disease or heart failure.[20] The GBS score has a better sensitivity in distinguishing high-risk patients who may need treatment from low-risk patients, compared with the Clinical Rockall score.[20] The Clinical Rockall score, which uses clinical data including age, systolic BP <100, presence of comorbidities, diagnosis, and stigmata of recent hemorrhage, is a better predictor of patient mortality compared with the GBS.[21] The AIMS65 score, which uses age, systolic blood pressure, mental status, INR, and albumin, is even more accurate at predicting mortality during hospitalization, as well as length of hospital stay and cost.[22]

There are few well-validated risk stratification models for acute lower GI bleeding. The NOBLADS-score (nonsteroidal anti-inflammatory drug [NSAID] use, no diarrhea, no abdominal tenderness, systolic blood pressure, antiplatelet use, albumin, comorbidity score and syncope), BLEED score (ongoing bleeding, systolic blood pressure, elevated prothrombin time, erratic mental status, unstable comorbid disease), and Strate score are models for predicting adverse events and mortality in lower GI bleeding.[23] However, inconsistent reliability and poor predictability have prevented widespread clinical use. A study performed by Ur-Rahman and colleagues investigated the use of the GBS in patients, with 1026 patients presenting with GI bleeding (562 patients with upper GI bleeding and 464 patients with lower GI bleeding), with primary outcomes being mortality, intervention, and transfusion.[24] The performance of GBS was similar in both upper and lower GI bleeding cohorts in predicting primary outcomes.[24] Although further research and evaluation are needed, this study raises the possibility that risk stratification models commonly used for upper GI bleeding, such as the GBS, may have clinical application in patients presenting with lower GI bleeding.

Approach to upper gastrointestinal bleeding management

The initial assessment of a patient suspected of having an acute upper GI bleed starts with a thorough history and physical examination. A rectal examination should be performed to identify the presence of melena or bright red blood. The use of nasogastric lavage in the setting of upper GI bleeding can be considered, but has a low sensitivity (42%-84%) and specificity (54% to 91%) for predicting upper GI bleeding based on 3 retrospective studies.[25] Additionally, there is a lack of randomized controlled trials studying the clinical benefits of nasogastric lavage.[26]

It is imperative that a thorough patient history include the timing of onset, any history of GI bleeding, use of NSAIDs, use anticoagulation or antiplatelet agents, history of liver disease, alcohol or tobacco use, and any risk factors for *Helicobacter pylori* infection.[27] Factors that are most relevant for identifying severity of bleeding include a history of malignancy or cirrhosis, hematemesis, hypotension, tachycardia, and a hemoglobin count of less than 8 g/dL.[28]

Early intravenous and transfusion resuscitation to correct hemodynamic instability, hematocrit, and coagulopathy in patients who present with upper GI bleeding has been shown to decrease mortality.[29] Early management should focus on correcting hemodynamic instability, hematocrit, and any underlying coagulopathy.

Red blood cell transfusion can be lifesaving in severe upper GI bleeding. A study of 921 patients who presented with severe upper GI bleeding compared a restrictive threshold for transfusion (hemoglobin <7 g/dL) against a liberal threshold (hemoglobin <9 g/dL); the results revealed less rebleeding, fewer adverse events, and a higher probability of survival at 6 weeks in the restrictive transfusion group.[30] Both the American College of Gastroenterology and European Society of Gastrointestinal Endoscopy guidelines recommend a restrictive threshold (hemoglobin <7 g/dL) as a target for red blood cell transfusion; however, higher hemoglobin levels may need to be considered in certain circumstances, such as for patients with known coronary artery disease.[3,31] The American Society for Gastrointestinal Endoscopy recommends red blood cell transfusion if there is active bleeding, significant blood loss, or cardiac ischemia, but does not identify a target threshold hemoglobin value.[28]

The use of proton pump inhibitor (PPI) therapy, such as omeprazole, pantoprazole, and others, in acute nonvariceal upper GI bleeding has become a mainstay of management. A Cochrane meta-analysis including 6 randomized controlled trials evaluated the benefits of PPI use before endoscopy revealed that PPI therapy treatment before endoscopy resulted in reduced high-risk stigmata of recent hemorrhage and need for endoscopic therapy.[32] However, there were no significant differences in mortality, rebleeding, or need for surgery compared with patients in the control group.[32] Additionally, another study found that scheduled PPI dosing and intravenous drip PPI therapy resulted in similar outcomes regarding mortality, length of hospital stay, and risk of rebleeding.[33]

A meta-analysis of the use of prokinetic agents in the setting of upper GI bleeding, specifically metoclopramide or erythromycin, demonstrated a reduced need for repeat EGD, but no significant impact on the number of blood transfusions, need for surgery, or length of hospitalization compared with placebo.[34]

Endoscopic management of upper gastrointestinal bleeding
Early endoscopy less than 24 hours after presentation in the setting of nonvariceal upper GI bleeding is associated with fewer blood transfusions and decreased length of hospitalization.[35] Endoscopy should be performed within 24 hours of admission once adequate fluid resuscitation and hemodynamic stability have been achieved.[27]

Table 3 displays the Forrest Classification, which is a tool that can be used to describe endoscopic findings of upper GI bleeding from peptic ulcer disease.[27]

Endoscopic treatment options for upper GI bleeding include injection, cautery, and mechanical therapy.

Endoscopic injection of normal saline or diluted epinephrine at the site of an actively bleeding lesion helps slow down active bleeding by causing a tamponade effect. Sclerosants, such as ethanolamine, pilodocanol, and ethanol, are other options for injection and work by creating tamponade and causing direct tissue injury resulting in thrombosis.[28] Sclerosants are not typically used in the setting of nonvariceal upper GI bleeding.

Cautery is another method used in treatment of acute upper GI bleeding. Thermal hemostatic devices, such as multipolar/bipolar electrocautery devices, heater probes,

Table 3
Forrest classification for describing endoscopic findings in patients with bleeding ulcers and predicting risk of rebleeding

| | Endoscopy | | After Endoscopy | |
| | | Rebleeding | | |
Forrest Classification	Therapy	%	PPI	Diet
I Active Bleeding				
Ia Spurting blood	Yes	55%	Intravenous[a]	Clear liquid[b]
Ib Oozing blood				Clear liquid
II Stigmata of Bleeding				
IIa Visible vessel	Yes	43%	Intravenous	Regular diet
IIb Adherent clot	Yes/no	22%	Intravenous	Regular diet
IIc Flat pigmented spot	No	10%	Oral	
III Clean ulcer base	No	5%	Oral	

[a] Intravenous PPI therapy twice daily should be continued for 72 h after endoscopic management before transitioning to oral PPI once daily.
[b] Clear liquid diet should be started immediately after the endoscopic procedure and then advanced as tolerated.
From Kamboj AK, Hoversten P, Leggett CL. Upper Gastrointestinal Bleeding: Etiologies and Management. Mayo Clin Proc. 2019;94(4):697-703. https://doi.org/10.1016/j.mayocp.2019.01.022.

argon plasma coagulation, and hemostatic graspers, can be used to achieve hemostasis in active bleeding.[28,36] Hemostasis occurs when heating tissue leads to edema, coagulation, vascular contraction, and activation of the clotting cascade.[36]

Mechanical therapy, such as an endoscopic clip or band, can also be used for obtaining hemostasis. During endoscopy, a clip is placed across a bleeding vessel and applies mechanical compression to achieve hemostasis.[28,36] A band is placed around a vessel or lesion in nonvariceal bleeding and helps to achieve hemostasis by causing compression, and tamponade is used to tamponade a bleeding area by direct pressure.[28]

A meta-analysis comparing different modalities for hemostasis in nonvariceal upper GI bleeding revealed the use of hemoclips is more effective at definitive hemostasis and reduced need for surgery compared with injection therapy alone, but there was no difference in mortality.[37] Hemoclips were similar in effectiveness to thermocoagulation in regard to rebleeding, need for surgery, and mortality.[37] A Cochrane Review found the combined use of injection with epinephrine and a second treatment option (no specific therapy mentioned) reduced the risk of rebleeding from 18.5% to 10%, emergency surgery from 10.8% to 6.7%, and mortality from 4.7% to 2.5% in nonvariceal upper GI bleeding.[38] The use of clips, thermal devices, and sclerosant therapy alone, or in combination with epinephrine, is recommended in patients with high-risk bleeding lesions.[28] Epinephrine is more effective than medical therapy, but is considered inferior to clips, thermal devices, and sclerosant therapy, and therefore, should not be used as a single therapy.[35,39,40]

Up to 24% of patients with nonvariceal upper GI bleeding may have rebleeding events despite the aforementioned treatment modalities.[28] If rebleeding occurs, repeat endoscopy is usually performed.[41] If bleeding is unable to be adequately treated via endoscopy, surgery and transcatheter arteriography and intervention (TAI) can also be considered and have similar efficacy rates.[42]

Upper GI bleeding from malignancies has a high rate of recurrent bleeding, ranging from 16% to 80%.[28] Although there is no optimal definitive treatment, options including surgery, angiography, and hemostatic powder are options for achieving hemostasis.[28,43]

Approach to small bowel bleeding management

It may be reasonable to consider repeating the upper endoscopy and colonoscopy to rule out a missed lesion, as studies have shown that upwards of 64% of suspected small bowel bleeding was caused by a missed lesion or source in the upper or lower GI tract.[44]

If a second-look endoscopy is planned, it is reasonable to perform a push enteroscopy. Push enteroscopy is a common method of evaluating the small bowel, using either an adult or pediatric colonoscope, or a dedicated push enteroscope that is approximately 250 cm in length.[45] The diagnostic yield of push enteroscopy ranges from 3% to 70%,[45] but despite this wide range in yield, it is commonly used for second-look endoscopic evaluation in suspected small bowel bleeding. The downside is that only approximately 70 cm of proximal small bowel beyond the ligament of Treitz is successfully evaluated, so complete evaluation of the small bowel is usually not achieved.[7]

Video capsule endoscopy (VCE) is a noninvasive diagnostic test whereby a patient swallows a pill that contains a small camera. VCE was first introduced around 2000, and can provide high-resolution images of the entire small bowel.[46] The VCE pill has a battery life of 12 hours and can take 2 to 6 pictures per second.[47] It is typically used in patients with suspected small bowel bleeding, Crohn disease, celiac disease, and small bowel tumors or polyps.[47] The diagnostic yield in patients with suspected bleeding is between 38% and 83%.[46] Once VCE reveals a bleeding source, another procedure, such as push enteroscopy, needs to be performed for therapeutic treatment. Approximately 86.9% of patients with an active bleeding source found on VCE had treatment that resulted in resolution of bleeding.[48] A complication is retention of the capsule, which occurs in about 2% of patients with suspected small bowel bleeding, and between 4% to 8% of patients with inflammatory bowel disease.[49]

Double-balloon enteroscopy (DBE) was developed in 2001, and uses an enteroscope with a balloon attached at the tip, and an overtube with a balloon that allows the scope to be advanced through the small bowel without looping.[50] DBE can be advanced from 240 to 360 cm beyond the pylorus, and 102 to 140 cm above the ileocecal valve with rectal intubation.[7] Compared with push enteroscopy, DBE can be advanced approximately 240 cm, allowing much more expansive evaluation of the GI tract.[51] The diagnostic yield for DBE is approximately 60% to 80%.[7] DBE allows for diagnostic and therapeutic intervention, such as the use of saline/epinephrine injection, argon plasma coagulation, hemoclipping, and tattooing for surgical resection.[52] Biopsies can also be performed via DBE.[52] Complications occur in approximately 3.2% of patients, with the most common being intestinal bleeding (1.3%), acute pancreatitis (0.9%), and perforation (0.2%).[53]

Single-balloon enteroscopy (SBE) is similar to DBE, but uses only 1 balloon located on the overtube. In a small study of 20 patients, the diagnostic yield was approximately 60% in SBE.[54] There are studies that show SBE has a similar diagnostic yield and therapeutic outcome compared with DBE.[55,56] SBE may also have a lower complication rate and might be safer in some patients compared with DBE.[57] Therapeutic options are similar to DBE.

Another technique to evaluate the small bowel includes spiral enteroscopy, which has a lower diagnostic yield of 57.1%.[58] Intraoperative enteroscopy, which requires a laparotomy, had a diagnostic yield of 80% in a small study of 20 patients,[59] but has a higher incidence of recurrent bleeding[60] and mortality of 17%.[7]

Small bowel barium radiography is no longer recommended for evaluation of suspected small bowel bleeding because of low diagnostic yield.[7,61] Computed tomography (CT) enterography (CTE) is another noninvasive method that can be used to assess for small bowel bleeding, but has a better diagnostic yield in overt bleeding.[62]

CT angiography can be used in the diagnosis of acute GI bleeding throughout the GI tract, with a sensitivity of 90.9% and specificity of 99%, and improved accuracy of the localizing the bleeding site.[63]

Approach to lower gastrointestinal bleeding management

The initial management of suspected lower GI bleeding should involve a focused history, physical examination, and laboratory data. A detailed inquiry into the patient's past medical history, medications, and any use of anticoagulants should be performed.[12] The presence of hematochezia with hypotension, as well as an elevated blood urea nitrogen (BUN):creatinine ratio greater than 30 should raise suspicion for a brisk upper GI bleeding source.[12,64] In patients who need resuscitation for hemodynamic stabilization, the use of intravenous fluids and blood transfusion thresholds should follow similar recommendations as used in patients with upper GI bleeding.[29,30]

Colonoscopy is recommended as the initial diagnostic procedure in lower GI bleeding, and is associated with shorter length of hospitalization.[12,65] However, there is evidence that suggests conservative management could be appropriate if the patient is hemodynamically stable.[66] The diagnostic yield of a colonoscopy ranges from 48% to 90%, and is both diagnostic and therapeutic.[12,67] Before colonoscopy, it is important to clear the colon via a bowel preparation to improve visualization and diagnostic yield, as long as the patient can tolerate a preparation.[12] Rapid bowel preparation strategies using a polyethylene glycol solution followed by colonoscopy within 24 hours led to improved diagnosis but no significant difference in mortality, length of hospitalization, transfusion requirements, ICU stay, surgery, and rebleeding.[68,69] Therefore, the optimal timing of colonoscopy remains an area of controversy requiring further research.

Colonoscopic hemostasis modalities are similar to those used in upper GI bleeding therapy, and include colonoscopic injection of epinephrine at the site of bleeding lesions, thermal hemostatic devices (eg, multipolar/bipolar electrocautery devices, heater probes, and argon plasma coagulation), hemoclips, and band ligation.[12] There are few data comparing the efficacy of each modality in the setting of lower GI bleeding, so the selected use of each method is based on bleeding location, access, and provider experience.[12] One case study of 137 patients with lower GI bleeding found that patients treated with hemoclipping achieved a 100% success rate compared with the other treatment modalities, as well as being safer than thermal contact.[70] Emerging techniques include topical hemostatic powders, which may be effective in controlling lower GI bleeding, but there have not been any randomized controlled trials performed, so data are lacking.[71,72] More comparative research is needed to further delineate which treatment modalities are effective, safe, and lead to better patient outcomes.

Radionuclide bleeding scans can be used in localizing a bleeding source, have a sensitivity of approximately 86%, and can detect slower rates of bleeding as low as 0.1 mL/min.[73,74]

Angiography is another procedure that is used in patients who are hemodynamically unstable and unable to tolerate a bowel preparation because of severe bleeding.[75] The diagnostic yield of angiography is about 40% to 78%, with bleeding rates of 0.4 to 1 mL/min required for positive results.[76] A meta-analysis found angiography with embolization was effective in 85% of patients with diverticular bleeding.[77] The rate of rebleeding is approximately 7% to 33%.[78] Bowel ischemia is a complication of angiography, and occurs in approximately 2.4% of patients.[79] CT angiography is a noninvasive tool that can be used to localize lower GI bleeding with a sensitivity of 85.2% and specificity of 92.1%.[80] CT angiography used prior to colonoscopy improves diagnostic yield by an additional 15% compared with colonoscopy alone.[81]

Surgery should be considered in acute lower GI bleeding if all other modalities have failed.[12] There is a reported 27% mortality rate in emergent total abdominal colectomy.[82] It is important to localize the bleeding site prior to surgery by using one of the previously mentioned diagnostic modalities to avoid unnecessary extensive resection or failure to resect the bleeding lesion.[12,78]

SUMMARY

GI bleeding is a common presenting complaint with an associated high morbidity and mortality. Although there is some research guiding clinical management of acute upper GI bleeding, more studies need to be performed to further delineate appropriate risk stratification of acute lower GI bleeding and compare treatment modalities.

CLINICS CARE POINTS

- Early resuscitation in hemodynamically unstable patients who present with upper GI bleeding has been shown to decrease mortality, and hemodynamic status should be optimized prior to endoscopy.

- When evaluating a patient with upper GI bleeding, the AIMS65 score, which uses age, systolic blood pressure, mental status, INR, and albumin, can be clinically helpful at predicting mortality during hospitalization, as well as length of hospital stay and cost.

- The use of nasogastric lavage in the setting of upper GI bleeding can be considered, but has a low sensitivity and specificity for predicting upper GI bleeding, as well as a lack of clinical benefit.

- PPI therapy treatment before upper endoscopy may reduce high-risk stigmata of recent hemorrhage and need for endoscopic therapy, but studies show no significant differences in mortality, rebleeding, or need for surgery.

- When caring for patients in the ICU setting, GI bleeding prophylaxis with a PPI should be strongly considered given the associated increased risk of mortality.

- Early endoscopy (<24 hours) in nonvariceal upper GI bleeding is associated with the need for fewer blood transfusions and shorter hospital stay.

- When treating acute nonvariceal upper GI bleeding, the use of epinephrine injection in addition to a second treatment option (thermal hemostatic devices, sclerosant or endoscopic clips or bands) reduced the risk of rebleeding, emergency surgery, and mortality.

- When evaluating for a source of GI bleeding and the initial upper endoscopy and colonoscopy or both, it is reasonable to consider repeat upper endoscopy and colonoscopy, as upwards of 64% of suspected small bowel bleeding cases are caused by a missed lesion or source in the upper or lower GI tract.

- When treating lower gastrointestinal bleeding, 1 study found endoscopic clips were more effective and safer compared with thermal hemostatic devices, but more comparative research is needed.

REFERENCES

1. Laine L, Yang H, Chang SC, et al. Trends for incidence of hospitalization and death due to GI complications in the United States from 2001 to 2009. Am J Gastroenterol 2012;107(8):1190–6.
2. Sey MSL, Yan BM. Optimal management of the patient presenting with small bowel bleeding. Best Pract Res Clin Gastroenterol 2019;42-43:101611.
3. Khamaysi I, Gralnek IM. Acute upper gastrointestinal bleeding (UGIB) - initial evaluation and management. Best Pract Res Clin Gastroenterol 2013;27(5):633–8.
4. Laine L, Jensen DM. Management of patients with ulcer bleeding. Am J Gastroenterol 2012;107:345.
5. van Leerdam ME. Epidemiology of acute upper gastrointestinal bleeding. Best Pract Res Clin Gastroenterol 2008;22(2):209–24.
6. Samuel R, Bilal M, Tayyem O, et al. Evaluation and management of non-variceal upper gastrointestinal bleeding. Dis Mon 2018;64(7):333–43.
7. Gerson LB, Fidler JL, Cave DR, et al. ACG clinical guideline: diagnosis and management of small bowel bleeding. Am J Gastroenterol 2015;110(9):1265–88.
8. Gerson LB. Small bowel bleeding: updated algorithm and outcomes. Gastrointest Endosc Clin N Am 2017;27(1):171–80.
9. Kuo JR, Pasha SF, Leighton JA. The clinician's guide to suspected small bowel bleeding. Am J Gastroenterol 2019;114(4):591–8.
10. Sakai E, Ohata K, Nakajima A, et al. Diagnosis and therapeutic strategies for small bowel vascular lesions. World J Gastroenterol 2019;25(22):2720–33.
11. Prakash C, Zuckerman GR. Acute small bowel bleeding: a distinct entity with significantly different economic implications compared with GI bleeding from other locations. Gastrointest Endosc 2003;58(3):330–5.

12. Strate LL, Gralnek IM. ACG clinical guideline: management of patients with acute lower gastrointestinal bleeding [published correction appears in Am J Gastroenterol. 2016 May;111(5):755]. Am J Gastroenterol 2016;111(4):459–74.
13. Strate LL. Lower GI bleeding: epidemiology and diagnosis. Gastroenterol Clin North Am 2005;34(4):643–64.
14. Targownik LE, Nabalamba A. Trends in management and outcomes of acute non-variceal upper gastrointestinal bleeding: 1993-2003 [published correction appears in Clin Gastroenterol Hepatol. 2007 Mar;5(3):403]. Clin Gastroenterol Hepatol 2006;4(12):1459–66.
15. Olsen KM. Use of acid-suppression therapy for treatment of non-variceal upper gastrointestinal bleeding. Am J Health Syst Pharm 2005;62(Suppl 2):S18–23.
16. Rosenstock SJ, Møller MH, Larsson H, et al. Improving quality of care in peptic ulcer bleeding: nationwide cohort study of 13,498 consecutive patients in the Danish Clinical Register of Emergency Surgery. Am J Gastroenterol 2013; 108(9):1449–57.
17. Speir EJ, Ermentrout RM, Martin JG. Management of acute lower gastrointestinal bleeding. Tech Vasc Interv Radiol 2017;20(4):258–62.
18. Toews I, George AT, Peter JV, et al. Interventions for preventing upper gastrointestinal bleeding in people admitted to intensive care units. Cochrane Database Syst Rev 2018;6(6):CD008687.
19. Mujtaba S, Chawla S, Massaad JF. Diagnosis and management of non-variceal gastrointestinal hemorrhage: a review of current guidelines and future perspectives. J Clin Med 2020;9(2):402.
20. Blatchford O, Murray WR, Blatchford M. A risk score to predict need for treatment for upper-gastrointestinal haemorrhage. Lancet 2000;356(9238):1318–21.
21. Rockall TA, Logan RF, Devlin HB, et al. Variation in outcome after acute upper gastrointestinal haemorrhage. The National Audit of Acute Upper Gastrointestinal Haemorrhage. Lancet 1995;346(8971):346–50.
22. Saltzman JR, Tabak YP, Hyett BH, et al. A simple risk score accurately predicts in-hospital mortality, length of stay, and cost in acute upper GI bleeding. Gastrointest Endosc 2011;74(6):1215–24.
23. Oakland K. Risk stratification in upper and upper and lower GI bleeding: which scores should we use? Best Pract Res Clin Gastroenterol 2019;42-43:101613.
24. Ur-Rahman A, Guan J, Khalid S, et al. Both Full Glasgow-Blatchford score and Modified Glasgow-Blatchford score predict the need for intervention and mortality in patients with acute lower gastrointestinal bleeding. Dig Dis Sci 2018;63(11): 3020–5.
25. Palamidessi N, Sinert R, Falzon L, et al. Nasogastric aspiration and lavage in emergency department patients with hematochezia or melena without hematemesis. Acad Emerg Med 2010;17(2):126–32.
26. Karakonstantis S, Tzagkarakis E, Kalemaki D, et al. Nasogastric aspiration/lavage in patients with gastrointestinal bleeding: a review of the evidence. Expert Rev Gastroenterol Hepatol 2018;12(1):63–72.
27. Kamboj AK, Hoversten P, Leggett CL. Upper gastrointestinal bleeding: etiologies and management. Mayo Clin Proc 2019;94(4):697–703.
28. Hwang JH, Fisher DA, Ben-Menachem T, et al. The role of endoscopy in the management of acute non-variceal upper GI bleeding. Gastrointest Endosc 2012; 75(6):1132–8.
29. Baradarian R, Ramdhaney S, Chapalamadugu R, et al. Early intensive resuscitation of patients with upper gastrointestinal bleeding decreases mortality. Am J Gastroenterol 2004;99:619–22.

30. Villanueva C, Colomo A, Bosch A, et al. Transfusion strategies for acute upper gastrointestinal bleeding. N Engl J Med 2013;368(1):11–21 [published correction appears in N Engl J Med. 2013 Jun 13;368(24):2341].

31. Gralnek IM, Dumonceau JM, Kuipers EJ, et al. Diagnosis and management of nonvariceal upper gastrointestinal hemorrhage: European Society of Gastrointestinal Endoscopy (ESGE) guideline. Endoscopy 2015;47(10):a1–46.

32. Sreedharan A, Martin J, Leontiadis GI, et al. Proton pump inhibitor treatment initiated prior to endoscopic diagnosis in upper gastrointestinal bleeding. Cochrane Database Syst Rev 2010;2010(7):CD005415.

33. Rodriguez EA, Donath E, Waljee AK, et al. Value of oral proton pump inhibitors in acute, nonvariceal upper gastrointestinal bleeding: a network meta-analysis. J Clin Gastroenterol 2017;51(8):707–19.

34. Barkun AN, Bardou M, Martel M, et al. Prokinetics in acute upper GI bleeding: a meta-analysis. Gastrointest Endosc 2010;72(6):1138–45.

35. Barkun AN, Almadi M, Kuipers EJ, et al. Management of nonvariceal upper gastrointestinal bleeding: guideline recommendations from the International Consensus Group. Ann Intern Med 2019;171:805–22. https://doi.org/10.7326/M19-1795.

36. ASGE Technology Committee, Conway JD, Adler DG, et al. Endoscopic hemostatic devices. Gastrointest Endosc 2009;69(6):987–96.

37. Sung JJ, Tsoi KK, Lai LH, et al. Endoscopic clipping versus injection and thermocoagulation in the treatment of non-variceal upper gastrointestinal bleeding: a meta-analysis. Gut 2007;56(10):1364–73.

38. Vergara M, Calvet X, Gisbert JP. Epinephrine injection versus epinephrine injection and a second endoscopic method in high risk bleeding ulcers. Cochrane Database Syst Rev 2007;2:CD005584.

39. Raju GS, Gajula L. Endoclips for GI endoscopy. Gastrointest Endosc 2004;59(2):267–79.

40. Stanley AJ, Laine L. Management of acute upper gastrointestinal bleeding. BMJ 2019;364:l536.

41. Lau JY, Sung JJ, Lam YH, et al. Endoscopic retreatment compared with surgery in patients with recurrent bleeding after initial endoscopic control of bleeding ulcers. N Engl J Med 1999;340(10):751–6.

42. Millward SF. ACR appropriateness criteria on treatment of acute nonvariceal gastrointestinal tract bleeding. J Am Coll Radiol 2008;5(4):550–4.

43. Leblanc S, Vienne A, Dhooge M, et al. Early experience with a novel hemostatic powder used to treat upper GI bleeding related to malignancies or after therapeutic interventions (with videos). Gastrointest Endosc 2013;78(1):169–75.

44. Zaman A, Katon RM. Push enteroscopy for obscure gastrointestinal bleeding yields a high incidence of proximal lesions within reach of a standard endoscope. Gastrointest Endosc 1998;47(5):372–6.

45. Raju GS, Gerson L, Das A, et al, American Gastroenterological Association. American Gastroenterological Association (AGA) Institute technical review on obscure gastrointestinal bleeding. Gastroenterology 2007;133(5):1697–717.

46. Rondonotti E, Villa F, Mulder CJ, et al. Small bowel capsule endoscopy in 2007: indications, risks and limitations. World J Gastroenterol 2007;13(46):6140–9.

47. Hosoe N, Takabayashi K, Ogata H, et al. Capsule endoscopy for small-intestinal disorders: Current status. Dig Endosc 2019;31(5):498–507.

48. Pennazio M, Santucci R, Rondonotti E, et al. Outcome of patients with obscure gastrointestinal bleeding after capsule endoscopy: report of 100 consecutive cases. Gastroenterology 2004;126(3):643–53.

49. Rezapour M, Amadi C, Gerson LB. Retention associated with video capsule endoscopy: systematic review and meta-analysis. Gastrointest Endosc 2017; 85(6):1157–68.e2.

50. Yamamoto H, Sekine Y, Sato Y, et al. Total enteroscopy with a nonsurgical steerable double-balloon method. Gastrointest Endosc 2001;53(2):216–20.

51. May A, Nachbar L, Ell C. Double-balloon enteroscopy (push-and-pull enteroscopy) of the small bowel: feasibility and diagnostic and therapeutic yield in patients with suspected small bowel disease. Gastrointest Endosc 2005;62(1): 62–70.

52. Otani K, Watanabe T, Shimada S, et al. Clinical utility of capsule endoscopy and double-balloon enteroscopy in the management of obscure gastrointestinal bleeding. Digestion 2018;97(1):52–8.

53. Nakayama S, Tominaga K, Obayashi T, et al. The prevalence of adverse events associated with double-balloon enteroscopy from a single-centre dataset in Japan. Dig Liver Dis 2014;46(8):706–9.

54. Vargo JJ, Upchurch BR, Dumot JA, et al. Clinical utility of the Olympus single balloon enteroscope: the initial U.S. experience. Gastrointest Endosc 2007;65: AB90.

55. Domagk D, Mensink P, Aktas H, et al. Single- vs. double-balloon enteroscopy in small-bowel diagnostics: a randomized multicenter trial. Endoscopy 2011;43(6): 472–6 [published correction appears in Endoscopy. 2011 Dec;43(12):1089].

56. Takano N, Yamada A, Watabe H, et al. Single-balloon versus double-balloon endoscopy for achieving total enteroscopy: a randomized, controlled trial. Gastrointest Endosc 2011;73(4):734–9.

57. Aktas H, de Ridder L, Haringsma J, et al. Complications of single-balloon enteroscopy: a prospective evaluation of 166 procedures. Endoscopy 2010;42(5): 365–8.

58. Buscaglia JM, Richards R, Wilkinson MN, et al. Diagnostic yield of spiral enteroscopy when performed for the evaluation of abnormal capsule endoscopy findings. J Clin Gastroenterol 2011;45(4):342–6.

59. Douard R, Wind P, Panis Y, et al. Intraoperative enteroscopy for diagnosis and management of unexplained gastrointestinal bleeding. Am J Surg 2000;180(3): 181–4.

60. Ress AM, Benacci JC, Sarr MG. Efficacy of intraoperative enteroscopy in diagnosis and prevention of recurrent, occult gastrointestinal bleeding. Am J Surg 1992;163(1):94–9.

61. Triester SL, Leighton JA, Leontiadis GI, et al. A meta-analysis of the yield of capsule endoscopy compared to other diagnostic modalities in patients with obscure gastrointestinal bleeding. Am J Gastroenterol 2005;100(11):2407–18.

62. Agrawal JR, Travis AC, Mortele KJ, et al. Diagnostic yield of dual-phase computed tomography enterography in patients with obscure gastrointestinal bleeding and a non-diagnostic capsule endoscopy. J Gastroenterol Hepatol 2012;27(4):751–9.

63. Yoon W, Jeong YY, Shin SS, et al. Acute massive gastrointestinal bleeding: detection and localization with arterial phase multi-detector row helical CT. Radiology 2006;239(1):160–7.

64. Srygley FD, Gerardo CJ, Tran T, et al. Does this patient have a severe upper gastrointestinal bleed? JAMA 2012;307(10):1072–9.

65. Strate LL, Syngal S. Timing of colonoscopy: impact on length of hospital stay in patients with acute lower intestinal bleeding. Am J Gastroenterol 2003;98(2): 317–22.

66. Moss AJ, Tuffaha H, Malik A. Lower GI bleeding: a review of current management, controversies and advances. Int J Colorectal Dis 2016;31(2):175–88.
67. Zuckerman GR, Prakash C. Acute lower intestinal bleeding: part I: clinical presentation and diagnosis. Gastrointest Endosc 1998;48(6):606–17.
68. Green BT, Rockey DC, Portwood G, et al. Urgent colonoscopy for evaluation and management of acute lower gastrointestinal hemorrhage: a randomized controlled trial. Am J Gastroenterol 2005;100(11):2395–402.
69. Seth A, Khan MA, Nollan R, et al. Does urgent colonoscopy improve outcomes in the management of lower gastrointestinal bleeding? Am J Med Sci 2017;353(3): 298–306.
70. Strate LL, Naumann CR. The role of colonoscopy and radiological procedures in the management of acute lower intestinal bleeding. Clin Gastroenterol Hepatol 2010;8(4). 333-e44.
71. Bustamante-Balén M, Plumé G. Role of hemostatic powders in the endoscopic management of gastrointestinal bleeding. World J Gastrointest Pathophysiol 2014;5(3):284–92.
72. Holster IL, Brullet E, Kuipers EJ, et al. Hemospray treatment is effective for lower gastrointestinal bleeding. Endoscopy 2014;46(1):75–8.
73. Leitman IM, Paull DE, Shires GT 3rd. Evaluation and management of massive lower gastrointestinal hemorrhage. Ann Surg 1989;209(2):175–80.
74. Smith R, Copely DJ, Bolen FH. 99mTc RBC scintigraphy: correlation of gastrointestinal bleeding rates with scintigraphic findings. AJR Am J Roentgenol 1987; 148(5):869–74.
75. Aoki T, Hirata Y, Yamada A, et al. Initial management for acute lower gastrointestinal bleeding. World J Gastroenterol 2019;25(1):69–84.
76. Eisen GM, Dominitz JA, Faigel DO, et al. An annotated algorithmic approach to acute lower gastrointestinal bleeding. Gastrointest Endosc 2001;53(7):859–63.
77. Khanna A, Ognibene SJ, Koniaris LG. Embolization as first-line therapy for diverticulosis-related massive lower gastrointestinal bleeding: evidence from a meta-analysis. J Gastrointest Surg 2005;9(3):343–52.
78. Davila RE, Rajan E, Adler DG, et al. ASGE guideline: the role of endoscopy in the patient with lower-GI bleeding. Gastrointest Endosc 2005;62(5):656–60.
79. Ali M, Ul Haq T, Salam B, et al. Treatment of nonvariceal gastrointestinal hemorrhage by transcatheter embolization. Radiol Res Pract 2013;2013:604328.
80. García-Blázquez V, Vicente-Bártulos A, Olavarria-Delgado A, et al. Accuracy of CT angiography in the diagnosis of acute gastrointestinal bleeding: systematic review and meta-analysis. Eur Radiol 2013;23(5):1181–90.
81. Nagata N, Niikura R, Aoki T, et al. Role of urgent contrast-enhanced multidetector computed tomography for acute lower gastrointestinal bleeding in patients undergoing early colonoscopy. J Gastroenterol 2015;50(12):1162–72.
82. Bender JS, Wiencek RG, Bouwman DL. Morbidity and mortality following total abdominal colectomy for massive lower gastrointestinal bleeding. Am Surg 1991;57(8):536–41.

Moving?

Make sure your subscription moves with you!

To notify us of your new address, find your **Clinics Account Number** (located on your mailing label above your name), and contact customer service at:

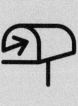

Email: journalscustomerservice-usa@elsevier.com

800-654-2452 (subscribers in the U.S. & Canada)
314-447-8871 (subscribers outside of the U.S. & Canada)

Fax number: 314-447-8029

Elsevier Health Sciences Division
Subscription Customer Service
3251 Riverport Lane
Maryland Heights, MO 63043

*To ensure uninterrupted delivery of your subscription, please notify us at least 4 weeks in advance of move.

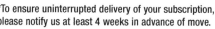

ELSEVIER

Printed and bound by CPI Group (UK) Ltd, Croydon, CR0 4YY

03/10/2024

01040480-0013